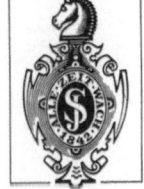

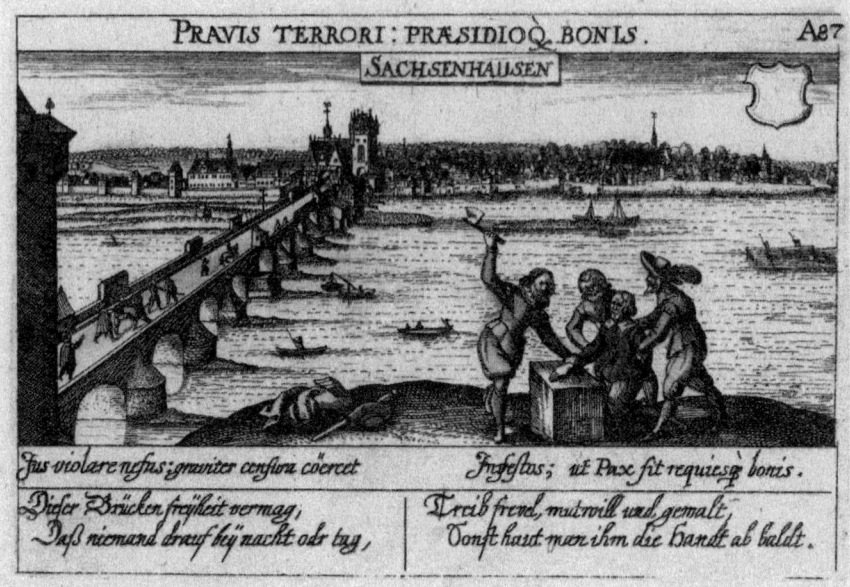

PRAVIS TERRORI: PRÆSIDIOQ. BONIS.

A87

SACHSENHAUSEN

Ius violare nefas; graviter censura coërcet   Infestos; ut Pax sit requiesq̃ bonis.

Dieser Brücken freyheit vermag,
  Daß niemand drauf bey nacht odr tag,

Treib frevel, muttwill und gewalt,
  Sonst hawt man ihm die Handt ab baldt.

Hans-Ulrich Steinau

Major Limb Replantation and Postischemia Syndrome

Investigation of Acute
Ischemia-Induced Myopathy
and Reperfusion Injury

With 42 Figures and 5 Tables

Springer-Verlag Berlin Heidelberg GmbH

Priv. Doz. Dr. med. Hans-Ulrich Steinau
Abteilung für Plastische und Wiederherstellungschirurgie,
Klinikum rechts der Isar, Ismaninger Str., D-8000 München

Translation: Susan Moore-Heidecke, München

ISBN 978-3-662-02482-9   ISBN 978-3-662-02480-5 (eBook)
DOI 10.1007/978-3-662-02480-5

Library of Congress Cataloging in Publication Data.
Steinau, Hans-Ulrich. Major limb replantation and postischemia syndrome.
Bibliography: p.
1. Extremities (Anatomy) – Reimplantation – Complications and sequelae. 2. Ischemia. 3. Muscles – Blood-
Vessels. 4. Surgery, Experimental. I. Title. [DNLM: 1. Extremities – surgery. 2. Ischemia – pathology.
3. Muscles – blood supply. 4. Muscles – pathology. 5. Perfusion. 6. Reimplantation. WE 800 S819m]
RD551.S69 1987 617'.58   87-26307
ISBN 0-387-15805-7 (U.S.)

© by Springer-Verlag Berlin Heidelberg 1988
Originally published by Springer-Verlag Berlin Heidelberg New York in 1988
Softcover reprint of the hardcover 1st edition 1988

2124/3020-543210

For Rita
who shared all the joy as well as the frustration,

and

for those patients who have endured the
agony of repeated limb loss

Preface

Posttraumatic stump formation and replantation of the severed limb are both reconstructive plastic operations which may lead to improvement or destruction of a patient's lifestyle.

For the primary attending surgeon, the difficult decision whether to undertake such an operation depends on the patient's clinical condition, the operational circumstances, the psychological and social aspects and, last but not least, on the surgeon's own abilities.

This monograph is designed as a synopsis of the great number of pathophysiological parameters and surgical and rehabilitational aspects which must be considered in the analysis of complications in major limb replantation. In addition, basic information about the key role of ischemic myopathy and microangiopathy is supplied, to encourage further experimental investigations.

As no new book is truly original, I wish to acknowledge the help of those listed below, with thanks for their friendly support, critical discussion, technical advice, and helpful cooperation:

Dr. A. Encke, Professor and Head of Department of General Surgery, University Hospital, Frankfurt, FRG;
Dr. O. Elert, Professor and Head of Department of Cardiothoracic Surgery, University Hospital, Würzburg, FRG;
Dr. E. Eriksson, Professor, Harvard Medical School, and Head of Department of Plastic Surgery, Brigham and Women's Hospital, Boston, Massachusetts, USA;
Dr. H. P. Fortmeyer, Ph. D., Director, Experimental Laboratory, University Hospital, Frankfurt, FRG;
Dr. M. Schneider, Ph. D., Department of Pathology – III, University Hospital, Frankfurt, FRG;
Dr. H. Förster, Professor of Biochemistry, and *Dr. Askali*, Department of Experimental Anesthesia, University Hospital, Frankfurt, FRG.
Ms. V. Beinrucker, HLM Laboratory, Department of Thoracic, Heart and Vascular Surgery, University Hospital, Frankfurt, FRG;
Ms. G. Schröder, Department of Surgery, Histological Laboratory, University Hospital, Frankfurt, FRG;
Dr. W. Haase, Institute for Numerical Statistics, Köln, FRG;
Dr. Bonhard, Dr. Uthemann, and *Mr. Boysen*, Biotest Inc., Frankfurt, FRG;

München, September 1987   Hans-U. Steinau

Foreword

The postischemia syndrome is of increasing importance in reconstructive procedures of the extremities. It is very likely that traumatologists and plastic surgeons will be confronted with local and systemic pathological reactions of cell necrosis and ischemia-induced microangiopathy in major limb replantation as well as with perfusion problems in pedicled or microsurgically transferred free flaps. The author therefore, analyzed the pathophysiological causes and the interactions of the developing "no reflow phenomenon" by reviewing an enormous number of references from the different subspecialities concerned. In addition, he presents experimental investigations on the value of oxygenation, substrate, and waste product transport during hypoxic conditions. The results show that perfusion with an oxygen-containing medium provides better prevention of the postischemia syndrome than the dry cooling preservation currently in use.

The author also describes the fact that in major limb reattachment, complications can become life threatening if there is no early intervention. Even in primarily successful cases ischemia-induced myopathy and microangiopathy impede the functional rehabilitation of the limbs. In the group of patients with large soft tissue defects, loss of flap requires complicated secondary surgical procedures.

This monograph fills a gap in its field, as the complex theoretical knowledge and the clinical and therapeutical consequences of postischemia syndrome have not previously been made a focus of attention.

I am proud that such an essential work has been prepared by a plastic and reconstructive surgeon, who has gained extensive experience in the prevention of possible early and late complications in replantations and flap transfers.

Munich, September 1987   E. Biemer

Foreword

Following animal experiments conducted since the beginning of this century, the first successful clinical replantation of a completely severed arm was performed by Malt and McKhann in 1962 on a 12-year-old boy. Since then further experimental work and the development of microsurgical techniques have moved replantation of large and small extremities into clinical practice. Yet technically successful replantations are still often endangered by infection, acute renal and pulmonary insufficiency, hypovolemia, and clotting defects. The most common causes of these complications are thought to be muscular ischemia and micro-angiopathy.

Hans-Ulrich Steinau, the author of this monograph, has contributed to our knowledge of the underlying pathophysiology by performing extensive animal experiments, which led to his "Habilitation" at the Johann Wolfgang Goethe University in Frankfurt/Main, and to his being honored by the German Surgical Society with the von Langenbeck Prize in 1985.

Steinau demonstrated that the perfusion of ischemic extremities, especially perfusion with an oxygenated hemoglobin solution, was significantly better at preventing the sequelae of ischemia than dry cooling.

Based upon the author's experimental work, extensive knowledge of the past and present world literature, clinical experience, and operative expertise gained in Frankfurt and Munich, this monograph gives an excellent synopsis of the pathophysiology of ischemic damage during and following the replantation of extremities. In addition to this critical survey, Steinau has added a chapter on the clinical importance of traumatic amputations of large extremities.

I am convinced that this monograph will be a valuable guide to all experimental and clinical surgeons who are interested in this field.

November 1987

Albrecht Encke, M.D.
Professor of Surgery
Johann W. Goethe University
Frankfurt/Main

Quotations to Note

Sir J. Hunter	– 1784	"Loss of a limb a man can hardly bear."
J. S. Haldane	– 1931	"Anoxia not only stops the machine, but also wrecks the machinery."
F. Griffith	– 1948	"Little good can come from attempts to relieve total ischemia of 12 hours' standing."
L. Koslowski	– 1959	„Durch isolierte Durchströmung geschädigter Glieder mit Hilfe künstlicher Herz- und Lungensysteme die Giftresorption aufzuhalten und auszuschalten."
R. Judet	– 1962	"Au niveau des membres, la vie c'est le mouvement."
J. M. Cormier	– 1962	"La mort est l'évolution fréquente en l'absence de l'amputation."
F. Linder	– 1965	„Darum kann gerade bei multiplen Traumen mit Gefäß-, Knochen- und Nervenbeteiligung auch heute noch immer der Entschluß zu einer Amputation weiser sein."
B. Mc O'Brien	– 1976	"Mild ranges of digital movement, combined with protection sensation, offer a better result than it is possible to achieve by a prosthesis."

Contents

1 Introduction

1.1 Historical Review

The desire to rejoin dismembered portions of the body appears recorded in holy legends as early as at the onset of the Middle Ages. Saint Eligius of Noyon (590 A.D.) is often depicted with the hind limb of a horse at his side, as he is said to have successfully replanted all four limbs of a horse (Eis 1956). There is also an account of Saint Hippolytus restoring the leg of an oxcart driver who had suffered the misfortune of losing his limb through a stroke of lightening. Yet another, similar case is cited within the Legenda Aurea: in the thirteenth century Saint Cosmas and Saint Damian are reported to have transplanted the leg of an unfortunate Moor to the stump site of a maimed Christian (Fichtner 1968). Interestingly, different representations of this very same replantation procedure can be viewed within three paintings. The Swabian masterpiece „Schnaiter Altar" (ca. 1500 A.D., Landesmuseum, Stuttgart) clearly portrays a proximal above-knee attempt, while the Spanish painter Fernando del Rincón (1600 A.D., Prado, Madrid) chose to present the situation as a distal above-knee procedure. A third depiction, produced by the Dutch artist Ambroise Franken, illustrates the leg being rejoined below the knee (1600 A.D., Königliches Museum, Antwerp).

The first concrete experimental replantation investigations reported actually date back to Höpfner (1903), Carrel (1906), and Guthrie (1912), who performed successful replantations of amputated canine hind limbs, though not without the frequent occurrence of septic complications.

In 1922, Halsted published his experimental findings on transplantation attempts he had carried out quite earlier, in 1897, involving canine hind limb neurovascular island grafts. According to his report, the formation of collaterals at the incision site 5 days postoperatively was so markedly intensified that severance of the main vessel was possible without necessarily promoting the risk of potential gangrene.

Among the first *clinically* documented cases of limb replantation was the successful revascularization of a subtotally detached upper arm performed by Jeger in 1912. Another such case was reported by Jianu in 1913 involving the amputation injury of a forearm that still possessed a subcutaneous tissue bridge. Replantation in both cases was accomplished by means of intussuceptional anastomoses. Within the same year Jianu also reported on his attempt at foot replantation following segmental limb-sparing tumor resection of a patient's lower leg. The procedure failed, however, due to thrombosis of the vessel anastomoses. Up to this point, his previous endeavours at limb replantation had been carried out solely on dogs, with a survival rate of up to 3 months.

Just prior to and directly following World War I, a great deal of investigative attention was focused on the conditions resulting from rhabdomyolysis, such as Volkmann's ischemic contracture, shock following crush/entrapment injuries, and subsequent renal failure (Frankenthal 1916; Hackradt 1917; Küttner 1918; Bayliss 1919; Cannon and Bayliss 1919; Colmers 1920; Minami 1923; Jepson 1926). In 1930, through the implementation of canine hind-limb strangulation studies, Blalock succeeded in disproving the theory that "toxic substances" caused tourniquet shock. He was able to demonstrate decisively that loss of plasma to the extremity was the triggering factor for the onslaught of tourniquet shock and that blood transfusions prevented the animals' death. In 1938, cooling of an extremity was introduced by Allen as a valuable therapeutic measure. A clear decline in mortality was observed in feline and canine models when the extremities were maintained at a temperature of 2° C during the ischemic phase. In 1942, the close parallels between tourniquet shock and the crush/entrapment syndrome were demonstrated by Duncan. He maintained that highly compressed hind limbs closely followed the same clinical course during the reperfusion phase as did strangulated hind limbs.

During World War II a still more significant contribution was made by Bywaters (1944) toward characterizing the postischemia syndrome, through the identification of marked hyperkalemia and ECG changes. He examined the pathological appearance of the kidneys following intravascular hemolysis and noted a significant decline in "pigment", creatine, and phosphorus, as well as the absence of glycogen within postischemic musculature. From these initial basic findings stem the rudiments of several therapeutic parameters still employed today in the detection and management of such conditions as urinary alkalization, the practice of extremity cooling, and the critical decision between fasciotomy or early amputation. Also during this period, a theoretical view on the tactical and technical feasibility of replantation utilizing *homologous* human limb members was presented by Hall (1944).

With the more recent experimental investigations of Lapchinski in 1960, the advantages of perfusing ischemically damaged muscles prior to replantation were clearly brought to the forefront. Following long-term phases of hypothermic conservation, amputated canine hind limbs demonstrated the ability to inhibit life-threatening circulatory, metabolic, and kidney dysfunctions, *provided* they had been previously flushed with oxygenated whole blood.

Finally, in 1962, the first successful replantation of a *completely* severed upper arm was carried out by Malt and McKhann 1964 in a 12-year-old male patient (Malt and McKhann 1964). This procedure took place more than 60 years following the first successful angiorraphy.

1.2 Statistical Frequency of Major Limb Replantation

In order to assess the clinical relevance and evaluate the operational organization of major limb replantation, the accurate accumulation of essential patient data is a basic requirement. While such an official source of exact information does not exist, it has been estimated that there are approximately one to ten cases of upper limb amputation per 100 000 inhabitants per year within an industrialized country (May and Gallico 1980). Similar figures have been published by the National Center for Health Statistics, presenting data for 43 000 major limb amputations during the year 1970 in the United States alone. Of these 43 000, only 25% were cases of traumatic mutilation (Friedman 1978). Another clinical poll undertaken by Ruby in 1978 produced an average figure of 6200 such accidents per year in the U.S.

In the Federal Republic of Germany the 1981 and 1982 Annual Reports of the *Bundesanstalt für Arbeit* (Bureau of Employment) presented representative data on this subject. During 1981, a total of 1451 patients were integrated into a government-sponsored employment rehabilitation program following traumatic extremity amputation. Of these persons, 90% were found to suffer more than 30% permanent work disability. Statistical data showed that 60% of the handicapped were unilateral lower-extremity amputees, while only 15% had experienced unilateral severance of an upper extremity and the incidence of bilateral lower-leg amputation was 10%. Interestingly, of the total number of victims, only 15% were female.

With regard to age, 80% of cases reported yearly involve persons under the age of 45. Despite this youth factor, only 40%–50% of these patients are deemed suitable candidates for limb replantation. Those found to be unsuitable are refused on the grounds of polytrauma, shock syndrome, or crush injury of the amputation stump or of the severed limb (Malt et al. 1972; Matsuda et al. 1978; Maurer et al. 1979, 1986; Berger et al. 1980; Chen et al. 1981).

The incidence of unusual replantation procedures such as extremity transposition in bilateral lesions, as well as stump preservation or distalization utilizing microsurgical transfer techniques, should also be integrated within the realm of replantation surgery (Sixth People's Hospital Shanghai 1967; Tsai 1981; Wang et al. 1981; Jupiter et al. 1982; Chen et al. 1982; Russel 1985).

1.3 Problematical Aspects of Major Limb Replantation and Prosthetic Supplementation

The undertaking of a major limb amputation confronts the primary surgeon with a decision of far-reaching consequences. The physician who chooses to follow the conventional and clinically accepted procedure of creating a functional amputation stump may harbor in the back of his mind the feeling that this course of treatment is mutilating, if not perhaps indicative of inability or a blunder on his part (Friedman 1978; Brown 1981).

The patients who have undergone such a procedure receive the shortest possible rehabilitation with a functionally suitable prosthetic device, but they also face the monumental task of psychologically adjusting to and accepting an altered body image. The stigma attached to a handicapped status will no doubt have a severe personal impact on their professional as well as their social future (Hoover 1964; Chaiklin and Warfield 1973; Marquart et al. 1976; Ruby 1978; Brown 1981; Beasley 1981; Florin et al. 1981; Hofmann et al. 1981; Stuhler and Schneider 1981).

Should the surgeon decide to go ahead with attempted limb replantation (provided the limb meets all or most of the required selection criteria), there is no absolute guarantee that this will lead to successful rehabilitation. Even in the instance of a technically perfect procedure with stringent therapeutic intervention and intensive perioperative care, there remains the potential threat of numerous complications. The following have been reported in the literature:

Mortality: Steinmann in McNeill and Wilson 1970; Kutz in O'Brien and McLeod 1976; Ferreira et al. 1978; Berger et al. 1980; Berger 1983; Baudet 1981; Coonrad and Milford 1981; Koch et al. 1981; Lee 1981; Lendvay 1981; Doi et al. 1983

Septic complications: Hardy and Tibbs 1960; Ramirez et al. 1967; Sixth People's Hospital Shanghai 1967, 1975; Denotter 1968; McNeill and Wilson 1970; Makris et al. 1973; Eger et al. 1974; Shaftan and McAlvanah 1976; Ferreira et al. 1978; Maurer et al. 1979, 1980; May and Gallico 1980; Coonrad and Milford 1981; Wang et al. 1981; Koch et al. 1981; Russell et al. 1984

Acute renal failure: Horn 1969; Harris and Malt 1974; Kutz in O'Brien and McLeod 1976; Maurer et al. 1979; Chen 1981; Koch et al. 1981; Berger 1983; Doi et al. 1983; Piza et al. 1983

Post-traumatic pulmonary insufficiency (ARDS): Inoue 1967a; Rosenkrantz et al. 1967; Berger et al. 1980; Jaeger et al. 1981; Koch et al. 1981

Severe hemorrhage and clotting disorders: Inoue 1967a; Denotter 1968; Halmagyi et al. 1969; Ely 1977; Matsuda et al. 1978; Meignier et al. 1979; Coonrad and Milford 1981; Hales and Pullen 1982

Thus, the surgeon should remain constantly aware of the potentially life-threatening postoperative complications that could come into play (multiple organ failure) as a result of major limb replantation. Following what initially appeared to be a successful procedure, he may in fact find himself questioning the sense of his original attempt to replant if numerous complications such as those listed above have arisen and the only option left is emergency amputation (Shaw 1963; Worman et al. 1965; Sixth People's Hospital Shanghai 1967, 1975; Ramirez et al. 1967; Paletta 1968; Chase 1970; Frank 1972; Chernov 1973; Eger et al. 1974; Morrison et al. 1977; Ferreira et al. 1978; Maurer et al. 1979, 1985; Berger et al. 1980; Koter et al. 1980; Jaeger et al. 1981; Koch et al. 1981).

Should the patient weather the acute danger period following such a procedure, there is always the possibility of primarily unforeseen circumstances such as chronic osteitis, ulceration, constant pain, persistent swelling, cold intolerance, frequent corrective surgical procedures, delayed functional improvement, or perhaps a permanent deficiency in functional limb capacity. Following months of therapy and treatment, the patient is both physically and mentally worn down to the point of perhaps doubting the success of the initial operation (Linder and Vollmar 1965; Paletta 1968; Jenny 1980). Probable loss of employment and the subsequent slide in social status, disintegration of the supportive family unit, and likely alcohol or drug addiction, carry a burdensome social stigma whose gravity can only be compared to that endured by an amputee.

Despite the obvious risk of potential complications, the decision to replant a severed limb is often undertaken rather than the alternative of amputation and subsequent provision with a prosthetic device. To understand the surgeous motivation are investigated the weak points and disadvantages of artificial limbs through a close analysis of their manifold uses. For this reason, the technical details and features of sophisticated prosthetic supplementation available today will not be addressed here; instead, a general evaluation will be made and problematical aspects will be discussed.

Whether a patient undergoes upper- or lower-extremity amputation, the agony of altered body image and body perception and behavioral reactions, beginning with initial denial, form a complex trauma. In addition to these burdens, there are somatic difficulties at the stump site through shearing forces and unphysiological pressure on skin and the soft tissues. Particularly in extreme climates, amputees suffer from allergies and infections, as well as from skin erosion resulting from excessive sweat production. The most serious sequalae, however, remain stump pain, phantom feeling, and phantom pain (Marquard 1966; Baumgartner 1973; Angliss 1974; Hofmann et al. 1981; Florin et al. 1981; Stuhler and Schneider 1981; Sherman et al. 1984; Krebs et al. 1985).

Along with the general hurdles already discussed, the intended functional purposes are often not completely met by a prosthesis. The upper extremities provide an extraordinary three-dimensional range of motion. At the distal point, the hand serves as a grip tool with highly sensitive pressure receptors. Sophisticated joint structures provide a complex spectrum of grip possibilities. Even in total darkness, complicated receptor and effector systems supply foolproof feedback on position, range of flexion, grip intensity, and texture and temperature of contacted objects. These senses, in unison with visual control and brain-directed motor function, combine to produce the complex feeling of body image. Prosthetic replacement of the upper extremities fails to satisfy amputees due to a lack of proprioceptive relay, diminished brain-directed motor function, and rejection as a part of the body (Baumgartner 1977).

A review of patients provided with a simple mechanical device during 1965/1966 by Ehrlich revealed that only 4% of unilateral, upper-arm or forearm amputees actually used the artificial limbs routinely at work. Even today, despite the clear advances in development of prostheses and specialized rehabilitation treatment available to amputation victims, statistics show that acceptance by the users remains a constant dilemma.

Long-term follow-up in cases of unilateral upper-arm amputated children showed that only 50% of the young patients finishing an intensive rehabilitation program actually utilized the provided prosthesis (Angliss 1974). For a similar group of youngsters Baumgartner (1977) reported an even lower acceptance rate.

In 1978 Vitali et al. investigated 263 consecutive cases of male adults who had undergone unilateral arm amputation. Of these, 62% never and 24% rarely wore their prostheses. Investigations concerning 53 female patients who had suffered the same fate uncovered even worse results: 94% refused the artificial limb completely and only 3.7% used it occasionally. Even the newest advances in rehabilitation therapy do not provide a complete solution to the problem of prosthesis acceptance, as has been pointed out in a study by Heger et al. (1985). In 678 cases of amputation collected from the recent literature, the average incidence of rejection for body-powered or electrically powered upper-limb prosthesis was 30%. From the remaining 70% success cases, 12% of patients actually rejected their artificial limb at a later time point.

Interestingly, in sharp contrast to unilateral amputees, bilateral amputees have proven to be the most accepting of all the patients. As early as 1966 Marquard published a report on his successful rehabilitation program in which ten of 17 patients routinely used their bilateral upper-extremity pneumatic prostheses more than 10 h daily.

Another preferred possibility for persons with distal bilateral forearm amputations is the formation of Krukenberg grips, which, following intensive rehabilitation, provide sufficiently sensitive and often unexpectedly good motoric function (Marquard 1975; Zrubetzky 1977; Friedman 1978; Baumgartner 1981; Kuhn 1982). Quite similar positive results have been achieved with the Sauerbruch self-regulated artificial hand. Through the creation of tunnels within the forearm flexors, movement capacity is transmitted to the prosthesis during self-willed flexion, while extensor function is provided by metal springs. Two thirds of the patients who had undergone this procedure (7–33 years post-op) continued to routinely use this simple prosthetic supplementation, according to a follow-up study carried out by Lang et al. (1982).

With the development of modern microsurgical tissue transfer, it has become possible to restore grip function through either transfer of a single toe to the osteotomized radius or combined transfer of a single second toe for use as a thumb with two-toe en-bloc transfer from the opposite foot to serve as fingers (Biemer 1984; Vilkki 1985). This operation not only offers the advantages of a highly sensitive and highly functional tool, but also provides the opportunity to wear cosmetically unobtrusive prosthetic gloves.

A clear improvement in the functional capability of artificial upper extremities is the employment of myoelectric impulses to direct the range of motion. Unfortunately, along with the advantages, there are still a wide range of disadvantages such as the lack of proprioception, limited use in dirty and heavy work situations, cumbersome and heavy models, intolerance to cold, and problematical repair service. The most basic problem surrounding prosthetic use remains the burdensome feeling of deficient body perception and the need for continuous visual control (Baumgartner 1977; Winkler and Baumgartner 1981).

The demands placed upon lower-extremity prostheses are not as sophisticated as those for upper extremities. Forward movement requires certain dynamically interrelated phases of stance, rolling, and swing elements. In contrast to the hand, the foot is not responsible for numerous complex and intricate functions; however, its capacity for extreme pressure and shearing forces is supplied through specified structures within the sole of the foot (Blechschmid 1932; Sommerlad and McGrauther 1978). The importance of innervated sole skin as well as the functionally integrated joints of the foot are essential elements in such functions as climbing, jumping, and running, and in the maintenance of balance over uneven surfaces (Clawson and Seddon 1960a, b).

The natural distribution of weight in human beings produces common difficulties at the stump site such as skin lesions and chronic pain. Of 178 unilateral, above-knee, young male amputees questioned by Florin et al. (1981), only 7%

claimed to live pain free, while 20% complained of intense or extreme pain up to 5000 h/year and an additional 30% reported 500 h of painful discomfort per year.

Two recent long-term follow-up studies by Sherman et al. in 1984 and Krebs et al. in 1985 showed evidence of up to 75% lower-leg amputees suffering from chronic phantom-pain symptoms. Though investigations have shown that these complaints may be triggered by a psychological defense mechanism against the trauma of limb loss, the somatic aspects of this dilemma should not be underestimated. Interestingly, a number of patients who have undergone stump revision and tenomyoplastic stump formation are permanently relieved of their misery (Davis et al. 1970; Marquard et al. 1976; Friedman 1978; Florin et al. 1981; Dederich 1981). Secondary revision itself has become a common event in hospitals with specialized rehabilitation programs for amputees, the frequency of such procedures averaging between 6% and 20% (Davies et al. 1970; Marquard et al. 1976). During his entire career, particularly in his experience with World War II veterans, Dederich (1981) claimed to have performed no less than 4600 amputation stump revisions to alleviate the problems described above.

One of the major points against major limb replantation is the argument that stump formation will result in earlier functional and social rehabilitation. This has been found generally not to be the case with patients who have experienced crush injuries of the lower extremities with subsequent guillotine amputation and open wound management. For approximately 2000 such patients, Davies et al. (1970) discovered an average interval between amputation and prosthetic supplementation of 5–6 months. Yet more data offered by Marquard et al. in 1976 showed that only 10% of their patients could be supplied with a lower-leg prosthesis within 4 weeks, while 25% needed 6–12 months and 29% required more than 1 year post amputation. Finally, correlating results were published by Kerstein et al. (1977) on 154 leg amputees who had achieved reintegration within an average of 19 weeks.

Once the patient has been successfully supplied with a functional prosthesis, the early rehabilitation program must be further supplemented with regular weight and gait training, along with frequent follow-up, in order to avoid the potential for imbalanced posture or perhaps even relapse.

Age presents still other problems, particularly as regards above-knee prosthetic supplementation with both children and older individuals. Young amputees will require either new prosthetic devices or alterations on a regular basis, due to the fact that they are still growing. Older persons, on the other hand, often reach the point where they are too weak to meet the "increased energy-cost expenditure" (Fisher and Gullickson 1978) of their artificial limb. For these patients the addition of crutches does not remedy the problem, and the end result is usually life in a wheelchair (Stuhler and Schneider 1981).

Along with the already described local complications, there is a controversial array of systemic disorders, perhaps correlated to the altered gait of the amputee. A common complaint is that of recurrent lower back pain brought on by stressful torsion, exaggerated lateral movements, and imbalances in weight und length distribution (Rompe and Nicthard 1982; Stuhler and Schneider 1981). Follow-up of 108 above-knee amputees showed an increased incidence of scoliosis and spondylitis of the lumbar spine, as well as coxarthrotic damage within the first 10 years following prosthetic supplementation. However, 16–20 years later, symmetrical alterations were observed (Breitenfelder 1981).

In the final long-term analysis, the basic disadvantages of artificial limb supplementation are clearly lack of proprioception, functional disability, deficiency of stump weight-bearing capacity, problems with repairs, chronic pain, intolerance to cold, and, finally, the psychological stigmata associated with the alteration in sociocultural relations.

Similar weighty arguments can be brought against major limb replantation. Though a successfully reimplanted limb may appear cosmetically attractive, complications such as hypo- and dysesthesia, dyshidrosis following neurorrhaphy (especially in the lower leg), skin ulcerations within areas of insufficient reinnervation, cold intolerance, and chronic pain may occur. In addition, high incidences of chronic osteitis, stunted growth from epiphyseal lesions in children, permanent functional loss, and socioeconomic disadvantages are potential risks that must also be taken into consideration (Woodhall and Beebe 1956; White and Selverstone 1956; Selverstone and White 1956; Clawson and Seddon 1960a, b; White 1969; Sunderland 1972; Seddon 1972; Kline 1980; Klammer and Schulz 1981; Omer 1981; Zwank 1981; Mumenthaler and Schliack 1982; Donski et al. 1984; Meyer 1984; Russell et al. 1984; Maurer et al. 1986).

2 Pathophysiological Analysis of Ischemia-Induced Injury in Major Limb Replantation

Ischemia, a term introduced by R. Virchow, is defined as the interruption of oxygen and subtrate transport to the cells in connection with the accumulation of degradation products related to stagnated flow within the tissue (Trump et al. 1976; Romanus 1977).

Tolerance of ischemia in severed limbs is closely dependent upon the possibility of compensation from related tissue groups. It appears necessary, therefore, to uncover the weak link within the chain and to analyze the pathophysiological mechanisms which may lead to decompensation and subsequent death of the replanted extremity.

2.1 Dermis and Subcutaneous Tissue

In clinical cases and experiments, the dermis and subcutaneous tissues have demonstrated a high tolerance for ischemia. Human full-thickness grafts, for example, following 4–5 days of storage at 4° C, demonstrate excellent take rates. Following 8–12 h of ischemia at room temperature, it was possible under experimental conditions in rats and rabbits to observe the first fat necrosis (Strock et al. 1968; Wilms-Kretschmer and Manjo 1969; Fuchs and Bodendieck 1975; Chait et al. 1978; May et al. 1978; Brunelli and Facchetti 1981; Weinberg and Song 1983). In 1982 Kerrigan and Daniel defined the critical ischemia time of 13 h in lipocutaneous island flaps in pigs, while earlier Milton (1972) had demonstrated a maximal time span of 10 h using a similar technique of occluding the vascular pedicles of island flaps.

When the clinically accepted procedure of hypothermia at 4° C was followed, rabbits and dogs developed initial intimal lesions following an ischemic period of 72 h (Donski et al. 1980 – rabbits; Tsai et al. 1982 – dogs; Schlenker 1982 – dogs).

Experimental investigations in large primates yielded similar results, e.g., with finger replantation in apes following 24-h dry cooling at 4° C without resultant dermal or subcutaneous necrosis (Hayhurst et al. 1974; Miller et al. 1979 a).

In 1977, Anderl reported the successful microsurgical transfer of a lipocutaneous groin flap in a patient following 30 h of storage at 4° C. A similar clinical experience was reported by Hentz (1981), whereby following 24 h of storage under hypothermia, a scalp flap was transferred without evidence of necrosis. As with clinical replantation of flaps, ears, and noses (Gibson 1965), good results can be expected with human peripheral limb replantation. The successful replantation of fingers and hand segments following more than 20 h of partial room temperature/partial hypothermic storage proves that dermis and subcutaneous tissue are unlikely to be hindering factors in human major limb replantation (Chen et al. 1981; O'Brien 1981; May 1981; Leung 1981; Biemer 1983).

2.2 Connective Tissue, Bone, and Cartilage

Results similar to those with minor replantations have been achieved with replants of connective tissue, bone, and cartilage. Albrektson (1982) was able to observe living bone cells within autologous bone graft despite 4–5 days of storage.

A clearly inferior tolerance threshold was present within the bone marrow of ischemic extremities of rabbits. Though cortical and cancellous bone structure maintained static function, reversible bone marrow lesions were observable following 15–60 min of ischemia (Schlagetter and Zimmermann 1956; Hübner and Zimmermann 1959).

Similar results were published by Berggren et al. (1982) and Östrup (1983), who employed microvascular rib graft transfers in canine models. Through hypothermic storage and simultaneous rinsing with Collins' solution there was a clear decrease in living osteocytes following the 4th h; however, osteoblast activity remained initially stable. Following 25 h of hypothermic storage total bone marrow necrosis was observed.

Experimental investigations into the influence of ischemia on the reunion of bones in replantation surgery produced delays in bone-healing processes within rat hind limbs following *12* h of ischemia (Kuwata et al. 1984). However, it appears most likely that ischemic destruction of the soft tissue was primarily responsible for the malperfusion of the distal femur, resulting in subsequent delayed healing. It remains to be further investigated whether long-term ischemia at room temperature has any direct relation to the frequent appearance of post-traumatic osteitis in major limb replantation (Zwank et al. 1980b).

Another potential problem with major limb replantation in children is the issue of growth plates. During experimental investigations involving juvenile guinea-pig hind limbs, Graf (Graf 1984; Graf et al. 1984) was able to demonstrate a retardation in longitudinal bone growth as well as increased destruction of the epiphyseal plates following a 2-h ischemic period at room temperature and limb replantation. Definitive conclusions pertaining to tolerance of ischemia in human epiphyseal growth plates are lacking, though various long-term clinical studies have reported findings similar to those obtained in other mammals (Furnas 1970; Streuli 1970; Nasseri and Voss 1973; Donski et al. 1984).

In view of stable static and mechanical function, as well as reversibility of histomorphological changes during clinically observed ischemic periods, bone, cartilage, and connective tissues have proven to be nonlimiting factors in major limb replantation.

2.3 Lymphatic System

Little information and few publications are available regarding the potential morphological and functional changes within the lymphatic system following ischemic injury.

In 1969, Willms-Kretschmer and Manjo reported observing lesions to rabbit skin lymphatics following 6–8-h periods of ischemia at room temperature, as well as following a 24-h postischemic phase. Endothelial walls of the lymphatics displayed obvious defects, a swollen endoplasmic reticulum, and cytoplasmic aggregations. Early lymphatic circulatory disturbances were indicated by intense dilatation distal to the stenoses.

Initial investigations carried out by Reichert, involving the recannulation of lymphatic vessels in experimental replantation, date back to 1926 and 1931. He reported findings of lymphatic vessel regeneration across the amputation site as early as the 4th postoperative day. From the 8th postoperative day, an efficient superficial and deep lymphatic drainage system could be seen. Similar experiences were reported by Danese et al. in 1962. Following severance of the lymph collectors, there were signs of sprouting collaterals reuniting on the 4th to 5th postoperative days. Fourteen days later, an unhindered lymphatic outflow from the extremity was seen. However, when a lymphangitis with subsequent obstruction of the lymph channels occurred, it was observed that subcutaneous lymphedema persisted. Comparable experiments performed more recently by Yong (1980) yielded similar results in a guinea-pig amputation model. On the 5th day following injury he observed sprouting lymphatic capillaries but significantly reduced regeneration of the lymphatic trunks.

In 1985, functional regeneration of once-severed lymphatics was made graphically clear by Kramer through the employment of radioactive tracers. As early as the 4th postoperative day, replanted hind limbs presented a resolution of diffused activity during lymph scans. The investigational team of Lanchow (1973) related finding a progressive regeneration of the lymphatic channels in canine models after the 7th postoperative day. On the 14th postoperative day, an extremely dense network of crossing lymphatics within the area of the amputation could be seen, similar to that observed in other animal models.

Another possible explanation for the gradual dissolution of lymphatic stasis following limb replantation was offered by Chachques et al. (1983). Using indirect lymphography and employing rhenium sulfur colloid marked with technetium 99m in a rat hind-limb amputation model, he concluded that, in addition to lymphatico-lymphatic spontaneous anastomosis, physiological lymphatico-venous communications were opened.

Regeneration of the lymphatics within the skin, subcutaneous tissues, and connective tissue sheaths of nerves, blood vessels, and tendons has been well established. However, the question of whether there is lymphatic regeneration within the musculature following replantation remains unclear, as to date only contradictory reports are available on the morphology of muscle lymphatics. Though it was possible for Aagard (1913) and Shdanow (1936, in Schroeder 1982) to illustrate an interfascicular lymphatic system within muscle through the injection of colored dyes, it was impossible for Adams et al. (1975) to confirm these findings within the endo- or perimysium. In 1974 Stingel found initial lymphatics localized close to the terminal venules but no evidence of lymphatics close to the muscle fibers or terminal arterioles. More recently, Skalak et al. observed lymphatics predominantly in the proximity of the transverse arterioles (1984).

In summary, ischemia-induced injury to the lymphatic system plays no significant role in terms of functional end results following major limb replantation. Even following periods of circulatory cutoff of greater than 8 h duration, no persistent interruption of the lymph drainage system could be seen when successful reconstruction of the dermis and subcutaneous tissues without circumferential defects had been achieved. Only postoperative soft tissue inflammation with destruction of the subcutaneous and perivascular tissue showed evidence of resultant lymphedema (Sixth People's Hospital Shanghai 1975; Chishueit 1975; O'Brien and McLeod 1976; Wang et al. 1981; Chen et al. 1981; Tamai 1982).

2.4 Peripheral Nerves

The determination of ischemic tolerance in peripheral nerve tissue is extraordinarily difficult, not only clinically but also in experimental investigations, owing to several potentially interfering factors. Pathophysiological conditions which cannot be avoided are:

1. Isolated ischemia of the nerve without circulatory disruption of the surrounding muscles
2. Compression lesions caused by the necessary utilization of a tourniquet
3. Secondary nerve compression brought on by compartment syndrome
4. Concomitant damage to the neuromuscular junctions
5. Interference of regenerational processes

In experimentally induced tourniquet paralysis of limbs, it was frequently difficult to differentiate between neurogenic lesions or muscle damage. As early as 1911, Bardenheuer described neurocompression lesions in cases of Volksmann's ischemia. He presumed that postischemic scar tissue formation led to an additional secondary process of neurodegeneration. Following 30 min of upper-arm tourniquet ischemia in human subjects, Castaigne et al. (1966) observed a decreased action potential and elongation of the latency period in arm nerves. However, they were unable to prove that nerve ischemia, and not tourniquet compression, was responsible for these changes.

Prolongation of tourniquet "ischemia" leads to a time-dependent increase in neurological deficits. Following a 4- to 6-h period of ischemia in canine hind limbs, Eiken et al. (1964b) was able to report severe contractility and conduction velocity disturbances. Quite similar changes were observed when a hind-limb tourniquet was applied to various other mammals such as rats (Bohn 1974), rabbits (Veicsteinas and Commande 1981; Brunelli and Facchatti 1981), and dogs (Hargens et al. 1981). Finally, in 1980, Rorabeck determined that a combination of ischemia and compression lesions was responsible for subsequent neurological disturbances which persisted for days following release of the tourniquet. Lower-leg paralysis with drop-foot position has been observed (Paletta et al. 1960; Rhea and Foster 1961; Shehadi et al. 1961; Martin and Paletta 1966) in cases for over a period of 12–14 days post-op (depending upon the degree of pressure applied). The paralysis seen was found to stem from morphologically identifiable changes. In 1972 Ochoa et al. demonstrated in primates a dislocation of the Ranvier nodes with partial or complete rupture of the myelin sheath at the tourniquet site. Further, a periaxonal edema within this region persisted for several months when ischemia was established through a pressure of 1000 mm Hg for 1–3 h at the level of the knee joint. Identical morphological findings of local demyelinization, as well as of fissures and vacuoles, have been reported by Lundborg (1970, 1982), Bradley and Thomas (1974), Thomason and Matzke (1975), Mäkitie and Teräväinen (1977 a), and Brunelli and Facchetti (1981) in varying species.

Within approximately the same time period Williams et al. (1980) showed through quantitative investigations in primates that a 25%–30% reduction in large myelinized fibers of the peripheral nerves occurred from tourniquet compression, with subsequent wallerian degeneration.

Through ligature of the aorta and femoral arteries in feline models, Korthals and Wiesniewski (1976) were successful in producing isolated segmental nerve degeneration without gangrene of the extremities. The resultant muscle dysfunction was so severe, however, that it was impossible to evaluate neuroregeneration potential following the peripheral limb ischemia.

Another troublesome dilemma involves the neuromuscular junction. Differentiation between ischemic lesions of the neurons or primary ischemic lesions of the muscle fibers with subsequent degeneration of the motoric end-plates is at present methodologically impossible. Initial structural changes of the motoric end-plates are observable in rats, rabbits, and dogs as early as 2–4 h following circulatory cutoff (Eiken et al. 1964 b; Dahlbäck 1970; Thomason and Matzke 1975; Mäkitie 1977).

With amputation injuries there is not only ischemia-induced damage to the end-plates, but also lesional insult due to severance of the supplying nerve fibers of the muscle cells (Josza 1976 a, b). It is therefore crucial that those who study degeneration/regeneration of the neuromuscular junctions in major limb replantation remain aware that lesions are the result of multiple factors.

Further investigations carried out by Lundborg (1975, 1977) on peripheral nerve ischemic tolerance levels produced evidence of a potential neuromicrocirculatory disturbance factor. He demonstrated in rabbit models that ischemic damage to the ischiadic and tibial nerves was reversible for up to 8 h. However, following more than 8 h of ischemia, deterioration of the blood/nerve barrier within the endoneural vessels did occur, with accompanying endoneural edema which blocked both the energy-dependent axoplasmatic flow and impulse transmission.

In 1980, experiments performed by Williams et al. in primates produced yet more significant insights. With a tourniquet at the level of the thigh and simultaneous compression of the lower calf for a period of 4 h they were able to differentiate between pressure-induced and ischemia-induced lesions.

When the results of investigations carried out by Mäkitie in 1977 are compared with those of Williams, it appears that a species-dependent factor may exist.

A staged 4-h period of ischemia in rat models produced longerlasting nerve conduction disturbances as well as more significant morphological damage than that observed in primate models. In the case of major limb replantation in human subjects, some published clinical reports maintain that sensory and motor function can be partially restored even following an extended ischemic period of more than 10 h (Chishueit 1975; Chen et al. 1981).

It was shown by Taylor in 1977 that an intact neuromicrocirculatory system is of vital importance to the speed of neurotization. There is, however, a lack of conclusive findings in the literature pertaining to the quantitative and qualitative influence of ischemic time on sensor, motor, and autonomous fibers, muscle, tendon, dermal, receptor, and Schwann cells, motoric end-plates, and finally, neuroregeneration potential.

Due to the numerous circumstances and dissimilar factors reported in the international literature, such as different amputation sites, varying range of age, coexisting injuries, diversified neurorrhaphy techniques, the presence of nerve gaps, and, last but not least, diverse rehabilitation programs, it is virtually impossible to establish a correlation between potentially ischemia-induced nerve lesions and functional end results following a major limb replantation. What can be concluded, however, is that ischemic damage to peripheral nerve tissue can occur under one or more of the following conditions:

1. Nerve ischemia resulting from primary circulatory interruption.
2. Nerve ischemia resulting from accompanying injuries with subsequent damage to the segmental vasa nervorum.
3. Nerve ischemia resulting from secondary compression injury within the compartment during the reperfusion phase.
4. Nerve ischemia resulting from scar tissue formation.

2.5 Ischemia-Induced Myopathy and Microangiopathy

2.5.1 Anatomical and Physiological Basis of Striated Muscle Perfusion

The provision of blood to the muscle is achieved through either segmentally or axially distributed major vessels (Legros-Clark and Blomfield 1945; Blomfield 1945; Mathes and Nahai 1982). Within the muscle, these two variations form a macromesh involving both arterioarterial and venovenous anastomoses (Spalteholz 1888; Stingl 1970; Duran and Marsicano 1979). The macromesh-originating blood vessels surround different groups of muscle fibers ("micromesh"; Krogh 1919a; Duran and Marsicano 1979), finally forming an ascending and transverse polygonal and (according to dominant fiber type) partially coiled capillary system (Hassler 1970; Stroinska 1979; Schröder 1982; Appel 1984; Groom et al. 1984). Contradicting reports have appeared concerning the number and distribution of capillaries for a single muscle fiber. It has been shown, however, that density of capillary distribution is dependent upon the demand of type-I (aerobic) or type-II (anaerobic) metabolism (Kunze 1969; Romanul and Pollock 1969; Eriksson 1972; Hudlicka 1973; Gray and Renk 1978; Gaudio et al. 1984). Plyley and Groom

(1975), however, argue that 3.2–4 capillaries per muscle fiber can be observed, irrespective of muscle-fiber type.

Within resting muscle, the supplying capillary system demonstrates zones of fluctuating hypoperfusion, that will be activated upon demand and called upon to carry out an additional nutritive function (Krogh 1919b; Zierler 1965; Tuma et al. 1975; Gaethgens et al. 1976; Grunewald and Sowa 1977; Honig 1977; Eriksson et al. 1983; Tangelder et al. 1984). It therefore appears that different capillary groups possess a permanent selective and even bidirectional flow pattern controlled by neurogenic and metabolic factors. Without these distribution mechanisms, the total muscular vasculature (which monopolizes 40% of the entire body) would be able to demand three times more cardiac output (Zierler 1965; Stock 1974; Messmer and Intaglietta 1986).

At the level of the arterioles blood flow is influenced by the following factors:

1. Changes within the transmural pressure gradient with adaptation of the myogenic tonus (Folkow 1964; Hanson 1964; Haddy and Scott 1968; Reneman et al. 1980; Tuma et al. 1975; Hellstrand et al. 1977)
2. Adrenergic vasoconstrictive (alpha) and cholinergic vasodilatative fibers (Brettschneider 1964; Skinner and Costin 1971; Hudlicka 1973; Johnson 1977; Duran 1979; Cain and Chapler 1980; Riede et al. 1981; Burnstock and Griffith 1983)
3. Metabolic products and changes in concentrations of: K^+, Ca^{++}, pO_2, pCO_2, number of H^+ ions, osmolality, kinines, lactate, ATP, vasoactive peptides, adenosine, substance P, and transmitter substances (Hanson 1964; Fairchild et al. 1966; Haddy and Scott 1968; Kontos 1971; Dobson et al. 1971; Skinner and Costin 1971; Barcroft 1972; Lundvall 1972; Scherer et al. 1973; Bockmann et al. 1975; Kawaramura et al. 1978; Duran 1979; Klabunde and Mayer 1979; Riede et al. 1981; Burnstock and Griffith 1983; Lindbom and Arfois 1984)
4. Tonus of the striated musculature (Groom et al. 1984)
5. Rhythmically fluctuating arteriolar calibers (vasomotion) (Groom et al. 1984; Lewis 1984; Tangelder et al. 1984; Messmer and Intaglietta 1986)

Controversy exists as to whether specialized precapillary sphincters are present within the wall of the arterioles, uniformly regulating the perfusion process (Hudlicka 1973; Chen et al. 1976; Dell et al. 1980). Experiments carried out by Hammersen (1965), Eriksson (1972), Eriksson et al. (1987), Fronek and Zweifach (1975), and Tuma et al. (1975) provided evidence that the smooth muscle fibers within the arterioles 20–40 μm in diameter are generally the regulators of peripheral resistance (Schmid-Schönbein et al. 1979; Lindbom et al. 1980).

At the level of the capillaries there are even more blood-flow regulating mechanisms:

1. The number of perfused capillary groups (Thulesius and Silvertsson 1973; Grunewald and Sowa 1977; Rhodes et al. 1978; Lindbom et al. 1980)
2. Frictional resistance of the capillary endothelium (Lacelle and Weed 1971; Schmid-Schönbein et al. 1979; Lindbom et al. 1980)

3. Blood viscosity, hematocrit, and configuration of blood cells (Suzuki and Penn 1966; Lacelle and Weed 1971; Brückner et al. 1971; Hudlicka 1973; Fuchs and Bodendieck 1975; Schmid-Schönbein et al. 1979)
4. Post-capillary venous reservoir (Eriksson et al. 1983)
5. Autoregulatory system of capillary hydrostatic pressures (Järhult and Mellander 1974)

From this list of parameters it is evident that oxygen and substrate supply to the muscle cells, as well as elimination of metabolic waste products, are regulated not only by flow rate, but also by the volume of capillaries involved within the process (Grunewald and Sowa 1977). Along these lines, it has been found that 1.35–6 ml blood/100 g muscle tissue/min is adequate to maintain metabolic demands in various mammals (Folkow 1964; Appelgren 1972; Eriksson 1972; Hudlicka 1973; Larsson and Bergström 1978; Grunewald and Sowa 1977; Moxley et al. 1978).

There are differing opinions as to the functional importance of arteriovenous shunts within the skeletal musculature. Using radiolabeled microspheres within canine models, Lopez-Majano et al. (1969) uncovered the presence of AV anastomoses along the entire length of the limbs. However, in similar experiments carried out by Spence et al. (1972) and Kennedy et al. (1981), individually scrutinized tissue groups within the limb were determined to possess AV anastomoses predominantly within the skin and subcutaneous tissue regions. Another investigation performed by Hammersen (1971) using dye injections provided evidence of AV anastomoses within the connective sheaths of the skeletal musculature. Due to their minimal presence and negligable shunt volume, these so-called bow capillaries appear to have no functional significance (Folkow 1964; Renkin 1971; Stingl 1971; Duran 1979; Kennedy et al. 1981; Myrhage and Eriksson 1984).

2.5.2 Regulatory Mechanisms of Fiber-type Distribution and Muscle Cell Morphology

During ontogenetic development the myoblasts differentiate into two primarily identical fiber types. Under subsequent neurotropic influence two essentially different multinucleated muscle fibers are formed, which can be identified and subdivided through complex investigational techniques (Guth and Yellin 1971). Perplexingly, more than six nomenclatures actually exist, according to species and methodology (Karpati and Engel 1968; Romanul and Pollock 1969; Dahlbäck 1970; Brooke 1973; Burke 1974; Buchtal et al. 1974; Eisenberg 1974; Gollnick et al. 1974; Adams et al. 1975; Khan 1976; Rubinstein and Kelly 1978; Bar-Or et al. 1980; Engel and Stonnington 1980).

The originally employed terms "red" or "white" fibers (based on myoglobin content) were found to be inappropriate in some species, while anticipated characteristics often did not correlate (Barnard et al. 1971; Khan 1976; Schmalbruch 1981). Therefore, in the pathophysiological considerations that follow a rough subdivision into two basic groups was chosen, based on the probability of reaction to complex amputation trauma and ischemic lesion (Hennemann and Olson

1965; Guth and Yellin 1971; Schmalbruch 1970, 1981; Gergely 1974; McGilvrey 1973; Karpati 1976; Artigue and Hyman 1976; Harrimann 1977):

Type I (red) — slow-twitch, predominant oxidative metabolism, energy source — triglycerides, delayed fatigue, high capillary and mitochondrial density

Type II (white) — fast-twitch, predominant anaerobic metabolism, energy source — glycogen, early fatigue, low capillary density

Though both fiber types can be found in all muscle groups, distribution is dictated by several functional principles (Bar-Or et al. 1980; Schmalbruch 1981). In 1965 Hennemann and Olson convincingly demonstrated this in feline triceps surae. The synergistic combination of the gastrocnemius muscle (predominantly type II) and the soleus muscle (predominantly type I) led to an optimal employment of accelerating reaction, maximal contraction, and continuous load capacity.

The morphology and distribution of mature fiber types remain under the influence of numerous regulatory mechanisms (Guth and Yellin 1971; Karpati 1976). In order to evaluate pathological findings within striated muscle, the following pathogenetic factors must be kept in mind, in as much as they create the potential for interference:

1. *Peripheral denervation:* generalized fiber atrophy (predominant type II) (Karpati and Engel 1968; Dahlbäck 1970; Erbslöh 1972; Bundschuh et al. 1973; Dorman 1973; Adams et al. 1975; Josza 1976a; Armbrustmacher 1978; Engel and Stonnington 1980)
2. *Chronic neuropathy:* fiber-type grouping, aggregated atrophy (Karpati and Engel 1968; Brooke 1973; Adams et al. 1975; Engel and Stonnington 1980)
3. *Partial paralysis:* generalized atrophy, increase in type-II fiber formation (Bundschuh et al. 1973; Brooke 1973; Brooke and Kaiser 1980; Burke 1974)
4. *Hypotony of the muscle:* type-I atrophy (Bundschuh et al. 1973) — diminished distinction between type-I and type-II muscle fibers (Josza 1976a)
5. *Decreased activity and/or lesion of the pyramidal tract:* type-II atrophy (Brooke 1973; Brooke and Kaiser 1980)
6. *Tenotomy:* type-I atrophy (Bundschuh et al. 1973; Brooke 1973; Hudlicka 1973; Wählby et al. 1978), tenotomy, and tendon transfer; varying atrophies with specific increase in type-I or type-II fibers (Castle and Rayman 1984)
7. *Varying levels of physical fitness:* massive variation in fiber type and diameters (Gollnick et al. 1974; Adams et al. 1975) — type-II muscle fiber hypertrophy (Armbrustmacher 1978)
8. *Immobilization, fixed joint deformity:* fiber types-I and -II atrophy (Guth and Yellin 1971; Karpati and Engel 1968; Booth and Kelso 1973; Jaffe et al. 1978; Brooke and Kaiser 1980) — increased variation in type-II calibers (Pongratz 1976) — degenerative fatty metaplasia and atrophy (Denzler et al. 1973)
9. *Arterial peripheral vascular disease:* focal fiber degeneration, relative type-I muscle fiber increase (Engel and Hawley 1977; Ängquist and Sjöström 1981) — type-I muscle fiber degeneration (Harrimann 1977), capillary fiber ratio changes (Clyne et al. 1982)

10. *Stimulation through increased or decreased frequencies, cross-innervation:* transformation from type I to type II or vice versa (Romanul and van Meulen 1967; Romanul et al. 1974; Guth and Yellin 1971; Erbslöh 1972; Brown et al. 1973; Dias and Simpson 1974; Armbrustmacher 1978; Dellon and Jabaley 1982)
11. *Venous insufficiency:* type-II muscle fiber atrophy and pathological fiber structures (Taheri et al. 1984)

Parallel to these histometrical and morphological changes, the skeletal muscle fibers will demonstrate metabolic and ultrastructual modifications as well. In experiments with animals it was shown that denervation of a skeletal muscle cell leads to intracellular reduction in contractile protein, along with a decline in amino acid, enzyme, and myoglobin concentration. Electron-optically it was possible to observe a reduction in the number of myofibrils in addition to a pronounced inability to take up blood-borne nutrients in the face of a vastly increased blood flow (Romanul and Hogan 1965). Coiling of the terminal vessel bed was also clearly seen (Hassler 1970; Stroinska-Kusiowa 1979).

During the phase of nerve regeneration following replantation, still another phenomenon could come into play. Under the influence of cross-innervation, long-term stimulation with an unsuitable frequency of another fiber type could result in a total change of enzyme patterns and in an increase or a decrease in supplier-capillary density (Romanul and Pollock 1969; Romanul et al. 1974; Myrhage and Hudlicka 1978; Hudlicka et al. 1984).

All in all, the skeletal musculature cannot be viewed as a totally static system. Even when there are only minute pathophysiological changes, a dynamic impact on basic structure and function can be observed. During the postoperative phase following amputation injury, ischemia, along with the previously mentioned factors, has an immense influence on resulting permanent muscular injury.

2.5.3 Muscle Cell Metabolism and Ischemia Tolerance

In contrast to the dermal, subcutaneous, and connective tissues, skeletal muscle cells have a higher O_2 and substrate requirement. In order for the cell membrane to carry out its task of transmembrane-potential formation (with the aid of active ion transport), stimulation, structure maintenance, and contraction activity, a stable and generous energy reserve must be available. The key metabolic substances are the energy-rich phosphagens. Among these, only ATP (adenosine triphosphate) is capable of creating energy through hydrolysis of the terminal phosphate group and thus converting it into the mechanical energy used in contraction activity and/or the electrical energy of the sodium-potassium pump (Gergely 1974; Enger 1977; Schröder 1982). Resynthesis of ATP occurs at different metabolic phases within the skeletal musculature (McGilvery 1973; Gergley 1974; Haljamae and Enger 1975; Fürst et al. 1976; Farber et al. 1981):

1. Within the mitochondria with oxidation of pyruvate, ketone bodies, and free fatty acids
2. With glycolysis to the point of pyruvate and lactate

3. With phosphokinase reaction
4. At high ADP (adenosine diphosphate) levels – the myokinase reaction

The major portion of energy synthesis, however, derives from the decomposition of triglycerides and glycogen/glucose (Jöbsis et al. 1979). The synthesis of energy-rich phosphagens is directly correlated to the oxygen supply level. For example, under aerobic conditions, the muscle cell is able to derive 38 mol ATP from 1 mol glucose. However, under anaerobic conditions, the cell can obtain only 2 mol ATP from the same amount of glucose (McGilvery 1973; Haljamae and Enger 1975). While the oxygen reserve within skeletal muscular cells is quite low (6–8 µl/g myoglobin) and the myoglobin storage system can maintain the regular O_2 tension only for a short time, the oxidative energy production is rapidly replaced by a less effective anoxidative energy synthesis. Access of the muscle cells to stored energy, as well as to available ATP and creatine phosphate (CP), results in approximately 22 fiber contractions. Following this phase, the energy supply must be guaranteed through anaerobic glycolysis (Keul and Keppler 1969; Karlsson 1971).

It may therefore be concluded that with amputation injuries, the complete interruption of O_2 and substrate transport, as well as obstruction of degradation product removal, leads to early cell storage depletion with a subsequent breakdown in cell function.

In addition, the intact original innervation of the muscle cell plays an essential role in the production rate of energy-rich phosphagens. In experimental investigations carried out in 1973, Brown et al. were able to produce alterations in oxidative and glycogenic enzyme patterns through continuous stimulation of the supplying nerve using unspecific frequencies. Similar experimental results were published by Hogan et al. (1965), Romanul and Hogan (1965), Romanul and van der Meulen (1969), Karpati and Engel (1968), and Telepneva (1973). They found (according to the dominant fiber type of the muscle) diminished synthesis as well as a slowdown in activity of the enzyme pattern following denervation.

Corresponding investigations in human subjects, performed in 1975 by Langohr et al., yielded similar findings, with decreases in glycogen and glycogenolytic enzyme levels predominating. It was in 1973, however, that Yakovlev revealed valuable insight into the role of the autogenous nervous system. He showed, that under induced work load following sympathectomy, an intracellular decrease in ATP concentrations took place in patients associated with a marked reduction in energy-rich phosphagen resynthesis.

Based on these numerous investigations, it is clear that severance of the peripheral mixed nerves will hinder recovery of postischemic energy production within the cell muscle.

Standardized parameters of cell pathology have been employed to investigate ischemia-induced lesions within muscle cells. Despite the fact, however, that most fundamental research that has been published pertains primarily to the cells of the parenchymatous organs, some of these criteria will be used with respect to the structural and metabolic differences for the skeletal muscular cell.

In 1958, Rotter defined the degree of ischemic lesion according to individual cell-component recovery time and thus introduced the term "individual vulnerability" (Rotter 1958 a, b). The muscle cell must be viewed as a complicated "multicompartmental system" (Leaf 1973) whose individualized functional components are crucially synchronized to assure well-organized performance. Any hint of adverse conditions will lead to a functional breakdown within the cell system. In the case of major limb amputation, long-lasting ischemia is directly responsible for a fatal vicious circle within the muscle tissue. Interruption of normal perfusion triggers within the muscle cells (after only a short interval) anaerobic energy synthesis, with a subsequent increase in acidic metabolites and a progressive depletion of glycogen stores (Stoner and Green 1948; Hofmann 1969; Kohama et al. 1971; Larsson and Bergström 1978; Hörl and Hörl 1985; Muramatsu et al. 1985). The increase in intracellular acidosis and hyperosmolarity is caused mainly by an accumulation of lactate (Hofmann 1969; Maeiwa et al. 1970; Keul et al. 1969; Karlsson 1971; Schnitzer and Stock 1973; Gebert et al. 1974; Stock 1974; Little and Reynolds 1976). These factors along with other simultaneously occurring disturbances of energy-rich phosphagen utilization, lead to a hindrance of the Na-K pump at the cell membrane. Parallel to these events, increases in intracellular Na, H_2O, and Ca occur, while K and Mg levels experience a rapid decline (Ravin et al. 1954; Fuhrmann and Crimson 1959; Kohama et al. 1971; Trump et al. 1976; Larsson and Bergström 1978; Dell et al. 1980; Jennische et al. 1982). As intracellular acidosis intensifies, a denaturation of the matrix enzymes within the endoplasmic reticulum takes place, as well as permanent destruction of structural protein synthesis (Trump et al. 1976; Farber et al. 1981). As a result of edema and permeability disturbances, mitochondrial function is reduced. It is assumed at this stage that precipitation of Ca and phosphate ions at the mitochondrial membranes is responsible for the resulting permanent damages (Jennings 1976; Romanus 1977; Farber et al. 1981). Finally, the liberation of proteolytic enzymes from ruptured lysosomes activates still another mechanism of intracellular lysis (Jennings 1976; Trump et al. 1976; Farber et al. 1981; Presta et al. 1981).

At the onset of the reperfusion phase the replanted extremity develops pathological concentrations (i.e., concentrations directly correlated to the severity of ischemic damage) of the following substances within the venous efflux:

Myoglobin (Bywaters 1944; Montagnani and Simeone 1953; Threlfall and Stoner 1957; Thompson et al. 1959; Rowland et al. 1964; Haimovici 1973; Biglioli et al. 1973; Kiessling et al. 1981)

Inorganic phosphate (Harmann 1949; Meroney 1955; Threlfall and Stoner 1957; Onji et al. 1963; Imai et al. 1964; Presta et al. 1981)

Potassium (Harmann 1949; Ravin et al. 1954; Dery 1965; van der Meer et al. 1966; Stock 1974; Brückner and Schmier 1974; Larsson and Bergström 1978)

Amino acids, purine bases, nucleotides (Macfarlane and Spooner 1946; Stoner and Green 1948; Green and Stoner 1952; Imai et al. 1964; Dery 1965; Deuticke and Gerlich 1966; Haddy and Scott 1968; Brückner et al. 1972; Hicks et al. 1980; Larsson et al. 1981; Schoenberg et al. 1985)

Enzymes (SGOT: Zimmermann and Springer 1966; Biglioli et al. 1973; Haimovici 1979), (LDH and isoenzymes: Zimmermann and Springer 1966; Wiesmann et al. 1969; Presta et al. 1981), (CPK: Wiesmann et al. 1969; Biglioli et al. 1973; Chiu et al. 1976; Presta et al. 1981; Quigley et al. 1981)

Acid phosphatase (Wiesmann et al. 1969)
Lactate (Harmann 1949; Lepage 1946; Karpf et al. 1973; Amundson and Haljamäe 1976; Enger 1977; Larsson and Bergström 1978; Miller et al. 1979 a)
Histamine-like mediators and proteolytic enzymes (Blaisdell et al. 1966; Massion
and Blümel 1971; Nakahara 1971; Pausescu et al. 1977; Hörl et al. 1982)

This weakening of physiological cell structure maintenance was defined by
Rotter (1958 b) as "postischemic cell membrane insufficiency."

Parallel to these intracellular factors, capillary permeability disturbances and
reactive hyperemia with an increase in capillary hydrostatic pressure resulted in
expanding intracellular and interstitial edema (Diana and Laughlin 1974; Thulesius and Silvertsson 1973; Welter et al. 1974). Edema formation, however, pro-
longs selected diffusion and transport pathways between capillary lumina and
subunits of the cells (Enerson 1966; Kunze 1969; Rhodes et al. 1978). Along with
this, there is another handicap while increased flow velocity of reactive hyperemia
abbreviates the contact time. In addition, destroyed intramitochondrial structures are rendered incapable of utilizing abundantly available oxygen concentrations (Stoner 1958 b; Karpf et al. 1973; Stock et al. 1974; Gaehtgens et al. 1976).

The following single or combined conditions will contribute to the irreversibility of a cellular ischemic lesion:

1. A decline in transmembrane potential and electrolyte shift (Koslowski 1959;
   Fuller et al. 1976; Jennings 1976; Enger 1977; Jennische et al. 1982)
2. A decrease in cell-volume regulation (Koslowski 1959; Enerson 1966; Leaf
   1973; Jennings 1976; Larsson and Bergström 1978; Dell et al. 1980)
3. Depletion of substrate and stores (Stoner 1958; Trump et al. 1976; Larsson and
   Bergström)
4. Intracellular acidosis (Stoner 1958 a; Trump et al. 1976; Kohama et al. 1971;
   Swartz et al. 1978)
5. Destruction of cellular subunits, membrane defects (Macfarlane and Spooner
   1946; Deuticke and Gerlach 1966; Leaf 1973; Baue et al. 1974; Romanus 1977;
   Larsson and Bergström 1978)
6. Abolishment of enzyme systems (Zimmermann and Springer 1966; Wiesmann
   et al. 1969; Biglioli et al. 1973; Jennings 1976)

Up to now it has been impossible to draw conclusions as to which of these factors is primarily responsible for the irreversibility of the ischemic lesion and subsequent cell destruction. It was maintained by Koslowski in 1959 that an insufficient energy supply is directly accountable for autolysis in muscle cells as well as
for a permanent imbalance of their metabolic system. A clear definition for critical ischemia tolerance time was offered by Deuticke and Gerlach (1966), it being
the point at which resynthesis of the lost nucleotides was still possible.

Some ten years later the term "point of no return" was introduced by Trump
to illustrate that even when cellular blood supply was restored, the ischemia-damaged mitochondria were unable to synthesize adequate levels of energy-rich phosphagens (Trump et al. 1976). Intracellular measurement of energy-rich phosphagens alone, however, can lead to false-positive readings of the cell system. A
decrease in transmembrane potential was found with intracellular potassium loss

in rabbit and human tissue at a period when no essential decline in ATP could be detected (Kohama et al. 1971; Romanus 1977; Jennische et al. 1982). It was assumed that this phenomenon was caused by blockage of the Na-K-ATPase activity by intracellular lactate acidosis (Kohama et al. 1971; Jennische et al. 1982). During postischemic reperfusion, however, intracellular ATP concentrations are a direct parameter for recovery of cell function, while the ischemic lesion of the cellular subunits leads to various periods of utilization deficiency of oxygen and substrate, as was demonstrated by experimental investigations by Stoner (1958 b), Karpf et al. (1973), and Stock et al. (1974). Corresponding data were collected by Romanus (1977), whereby a significant decrease of the ATP concentration within hamster cheek-pouch tissue persisted though sufficient oxygen and substrate were resupplied following a 4-h ischemic phase. Investigations utilizing canine hind limbs rendered similar findings. Following 5 h of tourniquet-induced ischemia, the muscle cells were incapable of synthesizing adequate levels of ATP during a subsequent 5-h reperfusion phase (Stock et al. 1974). Interestingly, inferior mammals such as rats have proven to be considerably more sensitive to ischemic lesions. Following application of a standardized hind-limb tourniquet for 4 h, the skeletal muscle in rats required more than a 4-week recovery period to initiate normal ATP synthesis (Bohn 1974; Swartz et al. 1978).

To clearly define ischemia tolerance one must also take into consideration that skeletal muscle is made up of varying fiber-type distributions. Slow-twitch (type-I) fibers, for example, possess an inferior ischemia tolerance but a superior malperfusion tolerance in comparison with other fiber types (Kaufmann and Albuquerque 1970; Jennische et al. 1979).

In conclusion, critical ischemia tolerance time, in terms of pathological criteria, can be defined as the duration of ischemia after which destruction of the cellular subunits results in a deficient production of energy-rich phosphagens, followed by subsequent death of the multicompartmental cell. This definition, however, proves to be clinically insufficient in relation to major limb replantation. First, striated muscle exhibits excellent regeneration potential; second, the organism as a whole is threatened early on by systemic phenomena of the postischemia syndrome; finally, the pathological damage to the supplying capillary system of the musculature must be taken into account.

2.5.4 The "No-Reflow Phenomenon"

During the clinical phase of the ischemic interval and reperfusion of severed limbs, cellular and capillary insults are seen that are due to a deficiency in oxygen and substrate, as well as to inhibition of degradation product elimination. The degree of damage observed is correlated to the duration of the ischemia, the ambient temperature, and the species type. All three factors determine the survival of the replanted limb.

As early as 1922, Brooks unexpectedly discovered and described the clinical symptoms of the "no-reflow phenomenon". Following a period of long-term arterial occlusion in canine models, he observed areas of focal malperfusion despite the presence of intensely pulsating arteries. Along with this, disseminated areas of muscle cell necrosis were found, which provided histomorphological correlation to his findings. Quite similar pathological changes following tourniquet ischemia in hind limbs were reported by Harman in 1948.

The term „no-reflow phenomenon" was formally defined by Ames et al. in 1968. First used in describing the initially zonal and subsequently total occlusion of ischemically damaged capillary systems within the brain, the term continues to be used today encompassing all tissues of the body.

Though development and severity of an ischemic lesion are dependent upon individual organ tissue vulnerability and type, the pathophysiological mechanisms that lead to subsequent malperfusion and cell destruction are the same. From a teleological point of view, the no-reflow phenomenon acts as a barrier to protect the uninjured remainder of the body from toxic products within the "dying extremity" (Blaisdell et al. 1978). As evidence for this direction of thinking, experiments performed by van der Meer (1966) showed a significant increase in the death rate of rats who had been administered heparin following 8–12 h of hind-limb tourniquet ischemia. In contrast to this, an untreated control group of rats demonstrated a higher rate of survival through the early development of the no-reflow phenomenon with dry gangrene of the affected limb.

It was shown by Strock and Manjo (1969a, b) in rat skeletal musculature that the no-reflow phenomenon is multifactorially activated. Such contributing factors are (see Fig. 1): hypoxia-induced swelling of the capillary endothelium, blistering and crease formations of the endothelial wall, vacuolization, endothelial rupturing, and disturbance of membrane permeability with venular leakage (Hammersen 1965, 1971; Bereiter-Hahn 1974; Fonkalsrud et al. 1976; Mäkitie and Teräväinen 1977a, b; Gidlöf et al. 1981; Brunelli and Facchetti 1981; Persson et al. 1985). As a result, severe stenosis of the capillary lumina will occur, potentiated by extracapillary factors. Traction of the connective tissue structures and compression of the capillaries through perivascular edema additionally reduce peripheral circulation (Strock and Manjo 1969a, b; Massion and Blümel 1971; Leaf 1973; Diana and Laughlin 1974; Welter et al. 1974; Gerbert et al. 1974; May et al. 1978; Lanz 1979). The factor most responsible for rapid postischemic edema formation appears to be hyperosmolality within the tissue along with postischemic reactive hyperemia, whereby blood flow of muscle tissue is increased up to ten times its level in resting conditions. Within the area of the already damaged terminal vascular bed, hyperperfusion leads to a rapid increase in the hydrostatic pressure gradient (Stock 1974; Diana and Laughlin 1974; Chen et al. 1976; Little and Reynolds 1976). Additionally, postdenervation supersensitivity of alpha-1 and alpha-2 adrenergic receptors appears to play a crucial role in rising peripheral resistance during reperfusion, as demonstrated by Clothiaux et al. (1985) with pedicled bone grafts and by Richards et al. (1985) with amputated rat hind limbs. Further, occlusion of the stenosed capillary bed is accomplished by embolization of hypoxically swollen granulocytes, erythrocyte and fibrin aggregates, thrombocytes, and endothelial fragments from major arteries (Hirsch and Gaehtgens 1965; Strock and Manjo 1969a; Willms-Kretschmer and Manjo 1969; Fuchs 1970; Fuchs and Bodendieck 1975; Brückner et al. 1972; Eriksson 1972; Karpf et al. 1973; Benner et al. 1975; Fonkalsrud et al. 1976; Little and Reynolds 1976; Romanus 1977; Mäkitie 1977; May et al. 1978; Bagge et al. 1981).

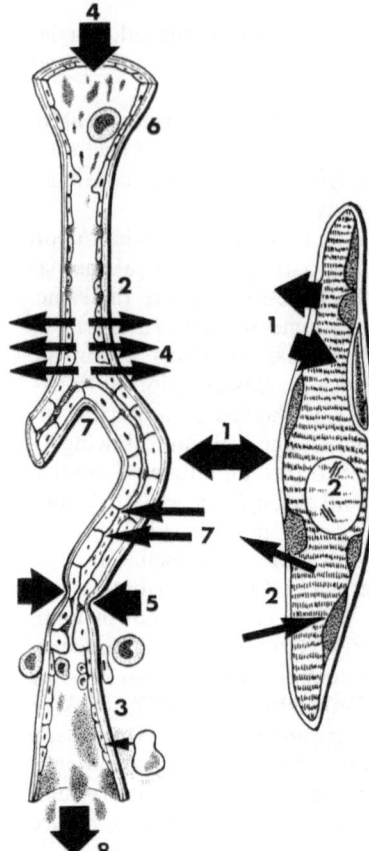

Fig. 1. Postischemic perfusion disturbances within striated muscle following major limb replantation; capillary system and muscle cell interaction.
1, Striated muscle cell exhibiting ischemia-induced myopathy, with membrane insufficiency, oxygen and substrate transport disturbances, and release of mediators;
2, secondary oxygen and substrate utilization disturbances resulting in destruction of subcellular structures, total loss of structural protein and enzyme systems, as well as in persistent membrane insufficiency;
3, thrombus formation, diapedesis, adhesion of thrombocytes and leukocytes to the venular wall mediators;
4, reactive hyperemia, edema resulting from hyperosmolality, massive increase in hydrostatic pressure, regulatory disorder in distribution of capillaries;
5, compression of the capillary through edema, enlarged cells, and intensified compartment pressure;
6, peripheral embolization from blood cells and aggregated endothelial debris;
7, decline in erythrocyte elasticity and inadequate washout effect along with capillary obstructuin;
8, flushing of degradation waste into the systemic circulation followed by "microembolization syndrome"

The remaining unoccluded capillaries show hindered oxygen and substrate supply and uptake as a result of increased blood viscosity and acidotic alteration of the shape of the erythrocytes (Brückner et al. 1971; Lacelle and Weed 1971; Fuchs and Bodendieck 1975; Schmid-Schönbein et al. 1979; Lewis 1984). In addition, pericapillary edema distends selected diffusion and transport pathways (Krogh 1919 b; Kunze 1969; Honig 1977; Grunewald and Sowa 1977; Rhodes et al. 1978; Shah et al. 1981). Increased flow reduction, contact activation of the thrombocytes through loss of endothelial basement membranes with exposure of the subintimal collagen, and activation of endothelial factors through degradation products of energy-rich phosphates lead to multifocal thrombus formation within the postcapillary venous bed (Gidlöf et al. 1979, 1981; Jöbsis et al. 1979; Matthias and Lasch 1981; Eriksson et al. 1983; Rosen et al. 1985; Stiegler et al. 1985).

The possibility has also been discussed that mediators released from hypoxic mast cells are responsible for endothelial lesions with subsequent thrombocyte aggregation (Strock and Manjo 1969 a, b). All of the contributing factors presented to this point lead to initially scattered areas of no reflow, finally affecting the entire capillary system with total perfusion breakdown.

Up to the present, it has been generally accepted that the previously described histomorphological findings and pathophysiological alterations during the post-ischemic phase were the *factor causing* the no-reflow phenomenon (Lewis 1984). However, evidence contradicting this view was offered by Eriksson et al. in 1983. His studies in the feline tenuissimus muscle paved the way to the differentiation between cause and effect of the no-reflow phenomenon. Through in vivo microscopy, the chronological development of postischemic perfusion disturbances could be observed. As early as 55 min following a 6-h period of induced ischemia of the muscle, scattered areas of obstruction within the postcapillary venules through platelet and erythrocyte aggregations were seen. Simultaneously to these findings it was observed that leukocytes and erythrocytes adhered to the endothelial walls and that diapedesis took place.

While the initiating mechanisms of these pathological changes remain unclear, several factors can be pointed to as possible instigators. One is the production of free radicals. These substances are normally synthesized intracellularly as by-products of regular metabolic pathways such as hydroxylation, peroxidation, and detoxification. In addition, stimulated macrophages (PMN) need oxygen free radicals in order to perform basic defense functions such as phagocytosis and inflammatory reactions (Freeman and Crapo 1982; Flohe and Loschen 1984; Rossi et al. 1985). It has also been discovered that several intracellular scavenger and competitive inhibitor systems protect the subcellular organelles and membrane structures from self-destruction. Some basic components of these systems, such as cytoplasmic superoxide dismutase (SOD-Cu-Zn), catalase, glutathione peroxidase (GPO), and mitochondrial SOD (Mn-Zn), along with the antioxidants cysteine, transferrin, ascorbic acid, carotenes and alpha tocopherol (vitamin E) serve as balancing substances (Del Maestro et al. 1980; Granger et al. 1981; Narayan et al. 1985). During the postischemic interval, low oxygen tension within the tissue is assumed to promote O_2-derived free radicals through univalent reduction of molecular oxygen. Numerous closely interrelated, complex destructive mechanisms are triggered by these highly active substances, which could explain the development of ischemia-induced muscle cell and capillary lesions:

1. Degranulation of lysosomes with subsequent release of proteolytic enzymes; plasmalemmal fatty acids such as arachidonate converted to peroxides (thromboxanes, leukotrienes, and prostaglandins) (Weissmann et al. 1979; Del Maestro et al. 1980)
2. Peroxidation of membrane lipids leading to toxic degradation products (Del Maestro et al. 1980; Kappus 1984; Risberg et al. 1985; Yoon 1986); degradation of hyaluronic acid, phospholipases, nucleotide cyclase, collagen, DNA (Granger et al. 1981; Kappus 1984).
3. Macromolecular leakage within the postcapillary venules (Del Maestro et al. 1980; Freeman and Crapo 1982; Ley and Arfois 1982; Proctor and Duling 1982; Gerdin et al. 1985; Bartlett 1986)
4. Catalyzation of amino acid oxidation, protein cross-linking and protein-strand scission (Freeman and Crapo 1982)
5. Leukocyte accumulation and adhesion by leukotaxis (Melmon and Cline 1967; Massion and Blümel 1971; Bartlett 1986)

As SOD, DMSO, catalase, GPO, allopurinol, soybean trypsin inhibitor, and sugar derivatives possess natural scavenger and/or inhibitor characteristics, they have been tested experimentally and clinically (Ley and Arfois 1982; Granger et al. 1981; Petterson et al. 1983; Gerdin et al. 1985; Im et al. 1985; Risberg et al. 1985; Shandall et al. 1985; Bartlett 1986; Húang 1986; Narayan et al. 1985; Yoon 1986).

As early as 1972, Brückner et al. inadvertently described the beneficial effect of allopurinol-hypoxanthine on dogs subjected to a 5-h hind-limb tourniquet; a significant decrease in edema formation was observed. He was, however, unaware of the substance's potential for oxygen free radical diminution and interpreted his results as increased resynthesis of ischemically destroyed cellular nucleotides.

There have been several *attempts* at accurate measurement of the effects of oxygen free radicals within different tissues in the past, but the literature available to date offers no proven *direct* method. Some of the procedures tried are listed below:

Bartlett (1986)	Macromolecular leakage and PMN accumulation, in vitro microscopy
Feng (1986)	Thiobarbituric acid color reaction as measurement of lipid peroxidation
Húang (1986)	Skin flap survival model
Yoon (1986)	Arachidonic acid metabolite, malondialdehyde (MDA)
Im et al. (1985)	Skin flap survival model
Narayan et al. (1985)	Spectrophotometrical assessment of enzyme activity in uric acid production
Risberg et al. (1985)	Edema formation, dry/wet weight ratio
Schönberg et al. (1985)	Hypoxanthine and xanthine production
Shandall et al. (1985)	Luminol-dependent chemiluminescense
Silin et al. (1985)	Superoxide generation: reduction of cytochrome-C as an index of superoxide anion
Chan et al. (1984)	Fluorescense microscopy leakage test
Petterson et al. (1983)	^{51}Cr-labeled erythrocyte trapping
Proctor and Duling (1982)	leakage, hamster cremaster pouch
Ley and Arfons (1982)	leakage test, Evan's blue
Granger et al. (1981)	Lymph-to-plasma protein concentration ratio, capillary permeability
Del, Maestro et al. (1980)	Hamster cheek pouch, leakage test

In general, the deleterious effect of oxygen free radicals deriving from ischemically damaged tissue cells and macrophages should remain hypothetical until a direct and proven method of measurement and assessment in muscle is developed.

Though it is not possible to list systematically the varying causes for destruction of the capillary bed, pathomorphologically it is most likely that the striated muscle cell is the base of the pathogenesis. The development and degree of post-ischemia injury vary within the different types of mammal tissue types. When compared, the experimental results of Ames et al. (1968) with brain tissue, Collins

(1969) with kidney tissue, Willms-Kretscher and Manjo (1969) with subcutaneous fat tissue, Leaf (1973) and Fabiani et al. (1976) with heart muscle tissue, and Cherry and Ryan (1976), Hallenbeck (1977), and May et al. (1978) with skeletal muscle tissue are proof of individual vulnerability. While there are no basic histomorphological differences between the capillary beds of the previously listed tissues, different specific metabolic functions of the "entity endothelium" are well known. Hemostasis and thrombosis, maintenance of membrane function, inactivation of humoral factors, repair and proliferation, receptor site for enzymes, and synthesis of prostaglandins and prostacyclins have been identified as typical endothelial duties (Hammersen and Hammersen 1985). It must be assumed that the individual cells of the endothelium and tissues possess their own specific reaction to ischemic lesion. During the reperfusion phase, the ischemically damaged "multicompartment system" (Leaf 1973) of these cells releases histamine-like substances, prostaglandins, lysosomal enzymes, proteinases, cell metabolites, and potentially oxygen free radicals, which together lead to the formation of the noreflow phenomenon. All of these factors are recognized as mediators in increased cell membrane permeability, cell wall disruption, pathological clotting mechanisms, and perfusion disturbances (Koslowski 1959; Hogan et al. 1965; Majno et al. 1967; Melmon and Cline 1967; Massion and Blümel 1971; Scherer et al. 1973; Schnitzner and Stock 1973; Baue et al. 1974; Pausescu et al. 1976, 1977; Grega et al. 1980; Amelang et al. 1981; Hörl et al. 1982). The general cell pathology and microangiopathy data presented to this point are illustrated in Figs. 42 and 43.

2.5.5 Regeneration Potential of Striated Muscle

To potentiate the assessment of persistent ischemic lesions within striated muscle fibers it is necessary to include evaluation of regenerational efficiency, which leads to recovery of function and cell integrity. Factors influencing the extent of ischemic damage are, of course, species, duration of ischemia, temperature, and fiber type. In animal experiments with dogs, rabbits, rats, and primates, the varying phase of reversible cell insufficiency stretching to the point of complete necrosis can be effected either through normothermic ischemia or deliberate induction of increased compartmental pressure (Zimmermann and Springer 1966; Thomason and Matzke 1975; Mäkitie 1977; Tountas and Bergman 1977; Brunelli and Facchetti 1981; Ludatscher et al. 1981; Mortenson et al. 1985). The regenerational processes reactivate, however, as early as 1–2 days thereafter. It was observed by Robert Volkmann back in 1893 that fiber regeneration took place principally according to the pathways of ontogenetic development. In the case of small intracellular defects, repair is performed by fiber-sprouting within the sarcolemmal sheath (Saunders and Sissons 1953; Kaspar et al. 1969, 1971). With larger defects, the differentiation potentials of surviving satellite cells and/or mononuclei play a crucial role as they infiltrate into or between the sacrolemmal sheath and fuse as myoblasts to multinucleated myotubes. At the same time, nomad monocytes that are present within the circulating blood invade the muscle cells, acting as macrophages by eliminating any existing fragmented necrotic sarcoplasma (Kaspar et al. 1969, 1971; Aloisi et al. 1973; Karpati et al. 1974; Engel and Hawley

1977; Mäkitie 1977; Chou and Nonaka 1977; Hall-Craggs 1978; Schmalbruch 1980; Carlson 1981; Schröder 1982). A battle for location is also taking place at this stage between the regenerating muscle fibers and the massively proliferating endomysial connective tissue producing fibroblasts (Constance 1955; Betz 1966; Adams et al. 1975).

At the primary stage of myoblast formation, intracellular polyribosomes induce the production of impressive amounts of contractile proteins. The influence of constant muscle tension and neurogenic factors govern the longitudinal direction of growth for the newly formed myofibrils within the multinucleated myotubes (Reznik 1970; Carlson 1973; Chou and Nonaka 1977). In animal investigations with rats and rabbits, generation of thin young fibers has been observed on days 10–18 following ischemic muscle necrosis (Le Gros-Clark and Blomfield 1945; Zimmermann and Springer 1966; Mäkitie and Teräväinen 1977c; Hall-Craggs 1978; Brunelli and Facchetti 1981). The first signs of end-plate regeneration within the anterior tibial musculature appeared in the rat on the 18th day post-op and on the 21st day post-op in rabbits (Allbrook and Aitken 1951). Without regeneration of the neuromuscular junctions, atrophy of the newly formed fibers resulted after the 21st day post-op (Wildbolz 1970; Carlson 1973; Hall-Craggs 1978; Schmalbruch 1980).

Despite the existence of regeneration potential, long-term muscle damage must be reckoned with in the face of long-lasting ischemia. It was pointed out by Zimmermann and Springer in 1966 that even 5 weeks after subjection of rabbits to tourniquet ischemia for 5 h, focal atrophy and fibrosis could be seen. Mäkitie and Teräväinen (1977) observed variations in caliber, split fibers, and centrally located nuclei 226 days after tourniquet ischemia (6 h) in rat hind limbs. Along with these permanent, mild-degree postischemic lesions, pathological conditions, including the possibility of muscle compartment mummification and calcification, could very well come into play (Horn 1969).

A factor essential to muscle regeneration is, of course, a sufficient supply of blood. This has been proven over and over again in free muscle transplantation without the benefit of vascular anastomoses (Faulkner et al. 1979; Carlson et al. 1979; Carlson 1981). While the outermost layers of fibers, nourished by perfusion, found it possible to regenerate, the inner portions completely necrosed and developed a secondary connective tissue replacement or fatty metaplasia (Lavine 1976; Carlson et al. 1979; Carlson 1981). Following free transplants of anterior tibial muscle in rabbit models, Kaspar et al. (1971) found that only 20% of the tissue survived. Some 8 years later, Faulkner maintained that only isolated muscle segments of less than 6 g had any chance of survival in transplantation. Therefore, the view offered by Robert Volkmann far back in 1893 that the replacement of skeletal muscle through free autologous muscle transfer is of no clinical value due to insufficient blood supply, remains valid today.

Histomorphological findings indicate the clear value of perfusion in terms of skeletal muscle fiber regeneration. One example of the benefits of perfusion is the accelerated phagocytosis of destroyed sarcoplasma within the proximity of the capillaries. Dense capillary proliferations, necessary in fiber regeneration, guarantee high levels of synthesis by providing increased quantities of O_2 and substrate transport. Following this intense phase of muscle fiber rebuilding, the density of capillary distribution returns to a more normal arrangement (Carlson 1973; Mäkitie 1977).

Unfortunately, up to now, it has been virtually impossible to accurately determine the beneficial role of regeneration potential in striated muscle in terms of major limb replantation in human beings. Interestingly, in experiments involving both inferior mammals and primates, the two groups followed almost the same morphological course during regeneration, despite markedly different ischemia tolerance levels. Human ischemia tolerance levels, however, are assumed to be even higher, which is attributed to the natural progression of the species. On the other hand, it is unlikely that regeneration following extended necrosis and calcification will occur, though isolated cases of actual regeneration have been reported (Horn and Sevitt 1951; Bütikofer and Mollegres 1968; Seddon 1966).

Definitive conclusions cannot be reached until the following questions have been answered through further clinical and experimental investigation:

1. At which point following an ischemic phase do the satellite cells and mononuclei lose their differentiation ability?
2. At which point during the ischemic phase are the sarcolemmal sheaths destroyed?
3. At which point during the ischemic phase does residual perfusion within the ischemia-damaged capillaries sink to the level at which regenerational process are no longer possible?
4. At which level of ischemic damage can it be assumed that capillary proliferation is inhibited?
5. At which point of the postischemic phase do scar tissue formation and fatty metaplasia supersede functionally efficient basic muscle fiber regeneration?
6. In the case of a poor functional end result, which factor is dominantly responsible: insufficient regeneration of the muscle cells or inadequate neurotization of the regenerated muscles?

Owing to a limited insight into these clinical problems, it must be assumed that ischemia tolerance time in striated muscle does not coincide with muscle cell necrosis. Neurophysiological data and metabolic cell assessments appearing within the literature are of no true clinical value, as major limb amputees are commonly revascularized following an ischemic period of more than 3 h on the average (Pennig and Brug 1982; Roder et al. 1985). Clinically, it is more important to closely examine (a) the influence of ischemia on the natural regeneration of striated muscle cells and (b) the significance of a surviving capillary system, which is vital to the restoration of residual function within the replanted limb. This *"critical repair phase"* in amputated limbs could be prolonged if a suitable perfusion procedure during the ischemic interval were undertaken, thereby avoiding life-threatening systemic complications during the reperfusion phase.

Another factor of clinical importance in major limb replantation is "secondary critical ischemia time". Following successful replantation, occlusion of the vascular anastomosis or development of a compartment syndrome can cause a repeat occurrence of ischemic damage to the limb, resulting in highly potentiated ischemic cell injury, as has been shown in experiments with isolated pig flaps (Kerrigan et al. 1984).

2.6 Compartment and Postischemia Syndromes

During the clinical phase of postischemic reperfusion, a surgeon should remain keenly aware of two potential pathological conditions which demand immediate diagnosis and surgical/intensive care intervention: compartment syndrome and postischemia syndrome.

2.6.1 Compartment Syndrome

The term "compartment syndrome" describes the development of localized muscle and nerve damage resulting from primary ischemic insult with subsequent pressure necrosis. Along with acute circulatory disruption associated with amputation injuries, the following conditions may also contribute to the perioperative development of compartment syndrome (Volkmann 1881; Colmers 1909, 1920; Jepson 1926; Mentha 1959; Seddon 1966; Bütikofer 1968; Mau 1969, 1982; Conner 1971; Ritland 1973; Gross 1978; Lanz 1979; Kingsley 1979; Halpern 1980; Matsen 1980; Renemann 1968, 1980; Quigley 1981):

1. Muscular contusions or fracture-dislocations
2. Delayed revascularization following embolectomy or vascular injury
3. Paravasal injection
4. Muscle edema following oppressive work load
5. Tourniquet, strangulating cast
6. Total circumferential burn injury of an extremity
7. Surgical procedures within the muscle compartment
8. Infection within the muscle compartment
9. Crush injury following entrapment
10. Pressure lesion due to hypotension during a period of unconsciousness (drug addicts, long periods under anesthesia)

During the reperfusion phase, any of the above listed clinical conditions will lead to intracellular and interstitial muscle edema. As the pressure within the fixed fascio-osseous compartments increases, the microcirculation within the capillary system is impeded. In the instance of major limb replantation, one major destructive force is the presence of increasing intracellular edema. This edema is caused mainly by ischemia-induced lactate accumulation with subsequent hyperosmolality of the fibers. In addition, a severe albumin-retensive interstitial edema occurs as a result of increased capillary permeability, an increase in total capillary surface, and an increased hydrostatic pressure gradient during reactive hyperemia (Moore et al. 1951; Hendley and Schiller 1954; Hewitt et al. 1971; Diana and Laughlin 1974; Stock 1974; Welter 1974; Little and Reynolds 1976; Hargens et al. 1978, 1981). Flow rates up to ten times the normal level can be seen as a result of acidic dilatation of the terminal vascular bed. Vessel wall smooth muscle is at this point ischemically distended and remains so through the influence of vasodilating cellular mediators and metabolites (Chambers et al. 1944; Fairchild et al. 1966; Dobson et al. 1971; Kontos 1971; Eriksson 1972; Stock 1974; Hellstrand et al. 1977; Duran and Marsicano 1979; Riede et al. 1981).

The duration and extent of reactive hyperemia is directly correlated to the level of oxygen deficit and oxygen uptake during the reperfusion phase. Through experimental investigations it was shown that tonal regeneration of the vascular system could be achieved within ischemically damaged muscle the instant that oxygen was added to the employed perfusion solution (Fairchild et al. 1966; Barcroft 1972; Stock 1974; Hellstrand et al. 1977).

Following ischemic periods of more than 4 h, the muscle compartments are more likely to develop a vicious circle: Expanding interstitial and intracellular edema hinder venous outflow and as a result, filtration pressure and malperfusion increases, contributing to yet more edema formation.

The significant role played by the venous section of the terminal vascular bed in edema formation was demonstrated by Pappenheimer in 1948. According to his findings, the postcapillary vascular bed is capable of producing the same amount of filtration fluid as that produced by the precapillary bed, using only one fifth to one tenth of the normally required pressure increase, however. The onset and extent of edema and the subsequent reperfusion injury can therefore be attributed basically to pressure changes at the venous portion of the terminal vascular bed (Lanz 1979; Reneman et al. 1980). These findings are in agreement with those reported by Su et al. (1982), whereby repeatedly blocked venous outflow in experimental skin flaps led to a higher incidence of tissue damage than blocked arterial inflow did. Therefore, it appears that an increase of pressure within the venous part of the capillary bed will have a much more deleterious effect on cell metabolism (Lanz 1979; Reneman et al. 1980).

The theory of "critical closing pressure" presented by Ashton (1965) maintained that vasomotoric occlusion of the arterioles took place when pressure levels dropped, resulting in subsequent collapse of the capillary pathways and abrupt breakdown of perfusion. Similar experiments carried out by Dahn (1967), Matsen (1980), Reneman et al. (1980), and Tangelder et al. (1984) did not produce results corresponding to those of Ashton, however.

Still another pathophysiological mechanism was proposed by Winninger in 1973. He suggested that the presence of retrograde flow within the AV shunts of the limb might be responsible for resulting pressure increases within the venous area of the vascular bed. Using radiolabeled microspheres, however, Kennedy et al. (1981) were able to illustrate that increases in shunt flow were only 8%–13% higher. Along with increases in pressure resulting from postischemic edema, obstruction mechanisms also come into play, as described in Sect. 2.5.4.

To avoid the possibility of partial or complete necrosis within the compartment, *early* operative revision is imperative. The surgical procedure must include fasciotomy of *all* involved muscle compartments of the limb as well as (in selective cases) subcutaneous displacement of the peripheral nerves (Peacock et al. 1969; Buck-Gramcko 1974; Lanz 1979; Nghiem and Boland 1980; Williams et al. 1980; Quigley et al. 1981; Mau 1982; Echtermeyer 1985). The proper time at which surgical intervention should be undertaken, from a clinical standpoint, is difficult to define. Although it may be possible to monitor a continuously palpable arterial pulse, this does not mean that the extremity is out of danger, since permanent muscle damage caused by expanding pressure within the venous area of the vascular bed continues to develop silently (Harmann 1948; Buck-Gramcko 1974; San-

derson et al. 1975; Adar et al. 1980). Such clinical symptoms as sensitivity disturbances within the deep branch of the peroneal nerve, limited range of motion,
pain with movement, and rising serum levels of muscle enzymes should be interpreted as signs of already existing damage. In clinical cases where the compartment syndrome is suspected, the only objective criterion available is continuous
intracompartmental pressure readings. In normotensive patients, intracompartmental pressure levels of 30–50 mm Hg are an indication for urgent fasciotomy
(Moore and Cardea 1977; Sheridan et al. 1977; Mubarak et al. 1978; Halpern and
Nagel 1980; Gelberman et al. 1981; Hargens et al. 1981; Wissing and Schmitt-
Neuerburg 1982). The value of prophylactic pressure readings within the compartments was investigated by Gelbermann et al. in 1981. They were able to show
that only 8% of patients who experienced 12 h of increased intracompartmental
pressure achieved complete restoration of normal limb function.

Along with surgical procedures, it has also been recommended that noninva-
sive treatments be given following the operation. One example is the administration of high-dose mannitol to decrease intracompartmental pressure (Shah et al.
1981; Hutton et al. 1982). Other nonsurgical treatments such as dry-cooling of the
extremity and intermittent application of external positive/negative pressure have
generally been found to be of no use clinically (Duncan and Blalock 1942;
Fuhrmann and Crisman 1959; Ashton 1975; Moore and Cardea 1977). What remains essential for the maintenance of perfusion are a constantly high pressure
gradient (monitored through frequent blood pressure readings) and the absolute
avoidance of limb elevation (Lanz 1979; Zweifach et al. 1980).

When intracompartmental pressures have not been released early, permanent
muscle damage must be reckoned with. If a limb has survived initial muscle necrosis and septic complications, it is common to observe such late sequalae as intrinsic minus deformities, Volkmann's ischemic contracture, or drop/club foot
deformities. Skin and subcutaneous tissue often fall victim to trophic ulceration
and chronic paronychia owing to disturbances in blood flow distribution and peripheral nerve lesions (Sixth People's Hospital Shanghai 1967, 1975; Morton et
al. 1969; Peacock et al. 1969; Maurer et al. 1979; May and Gallico 1980; Reneman
et al. 1980; Mau 1982; Meyer 1984; Russell et al. 1984).

During the phase of postischemic reperfusion following major limb replantation, intensive care must include constant measurement of intracompartmental
pressures. With *normothermic* ischemia of more than 4 h duration, primary
fasciotomy is clearly indicated. Early release of intracompartmental pressures not
only results in immediate improvement of oxygen and substrate supply, but also
guarantees an adequate level of perfusion for regenerating fibers.

2.6.2 Postischemia Syndrome

In sharp contrast to limited area compartment syndrome, normothermic ischemic
periods of more than 4 h affecting large areas of muscle present the potential development of life-threatening complications. In cases where major limb parts are
involved, the influx of muscular waste products into other organs of the body
could very well lead to a fatal outcome.

Depending upon the causal circumstances surrounding the development of postischemia syndrome, different terms such as tourniquet, crush, compression, myonephropathic-metabolic, and Legrain-Courmier syndrome are commonly used (Küttner 1818; Bayliss 1919; Cannon and Bayliss 1919; Blalock 1930; Duran and Blalock 1942; Bywaters 1944; Linder and Vollmar 1965; Weeks 1968; Haimovici 1973, 1979; Larcan et al. 1973; Marty 1973; Love 1978; Santangelo et al. 1982). The onset of postischemia syndrome, however, is feared not only in major limb replantation, but also with the following clinical situations:

1. Late revascularization following injury to a major artery or embolization
2. Entrapment or crush injury
3. Tourniquet ischemia of more than 4 h duration
4. Strangulating casts
5. Total circumferential burn injury of an extremity
6. Development of pressure lesion following a period of unconsciousness

Clinical cases have shown a clear correlation between duration of ischemia and the incidence of severe complications. In a report by Miller in 1949, the amputation rate for patients suffering injuries to the major arteries during World War II ranged between 30% and 70%. The amelioration of conditions for surgery during the subsequent wars in Korea and Vietnam lowered the frequency of amputations to between 13% and 20% (Hughes 1958; Chandler and Knapp 1967). Finally, during the more recent Middle East conflicts, amputation rates dropped to 7% in patients with comparable lesions of their major limb arteries. This obvious decrease in the incidence of required amputation can be directly attributed to a reduction in the ischemic interval (Adar et al. 1980).

Oddly enough, reported cases of amputation are rising today, as lesions to major arteries are not recognized soon enough. Blunt injuries to the popliteal artery followed by second-stage thrombotic occlusion has been associated with amputation rates of 24%–50% due to prolonged ischemic periods (Johanson et al. 1982; Snyder 1982). Along with the grievous loss of a limb, postischemia syndrome following delayed revascularization also contributes to a marked increase in mortality (Cormier and Legrain 1962; Cormier and Devin 1969; Larcan et al. 1973; Haimovici 1973, 1979; Denck et al. 1977; Abbott et al. 1982). For this reason it is recommended that limbs subjected to complete normothermic ischemia for more than 10 h be amputated, to avoid exposing the remainder of the body to possibly life-threatening complications (Bywaters 1944; Eigler 1974; Kindhäuser and Eigler 1980). A clear example of the threat posed by the development of postischemia syndrome was given by Steinmann (McNeil and Wilson 1970); subsequent to upper-arm replantation (following a 3.5-h warm ischemic period) the patient died of post-ischemia-related complications. Another case was reported by Inoue (1967 b), in which a patient developed acute cardiac arrest following replantation, although the reestablished upper arm had previously been stored for 7 h under partially hypothermic conditions.

From all of the presented experimental and clinical data pertaining to the postischemia syndrome, it is clear that this condition has the potential for leading to multiple organ failure (MOF) and possibly death (Doi et al. 1983).

2.6.2.1 Circulatory System and Metabolic Disorders

Once the reattachment of a severed limb is accomplished the "declamping phe-nomenon" will follow, characterized by a massive drop in blood pressure and a significant decline in total peripheral resistence. Observed as well are compensa-tory increases in the heart and respiratory rates and in respiratory total volume. An expanding sequestration of plasma within the ischemically damaged extremity leads to severe hemoconcentration throughout the remainder of the body (Saar 1913; Cannon and Bayljss 1919; Blalock 1930; Bywaters 1944; Kristen et al. 1970; Stock 1974). In animal experiments where hind-limb tourniquets were applied, the loss of plasma to the affected extremity averaged 1%–7.5% of total body weight, depending upon the duration of ischemia, the temperature, and the amount of muscle mass involved. This tourniquet method is commonly used in dog and rat experimental models to produce standardized volume-deficiency shock (Wilson and Roome 1936; Schwiegk 1942; Duncan and Blalock 1942; Kety et al. 1945; Nathanson et al. 1945; Koletsky and Klein 1955; van der Meer et al. 1966; Hoffmann 1969). Experimental procedures with bilateral rabbit hind-limb tourniquets carried out by Little and Reynolds in 1976 produced a total edema formation of 56% within the first 10 min of restored perfusion to the limbs. The pathophysiological mechanisms responsible for this fluid sequestration have been established as ischemic tissue hyperosmolality, reactive hyperemia with a sub-sequent increase in pressure gradient, and permeability disturbances of the capil-lary system. Parallel to these events, a significant washout of potassium and acidic metabolites from the ischemic extremity can be also detected. Venous runoff samples collected during various experiments (Kristen et al. 1970; Brückner et al. 1971) have revealed systemic potassium levels as high as 14 mEq/l, while Stock (1974) reported values of 7.88 mEq/l within aortic blood. During the end stage of experiments with rats, van der Meer et al. (1966) discovered potassium levels of 10–13 mEq within arterial blood samples. In addition to these findings, during the initial reperfusion phase a severe decrease in systemic pH to a level of 7.1 and a rise in hematocrit up to 70% were observed in canine hind-limb models that had previously undergone 5–7 h of tourniquet ischemia (Paul et al. 1965; Brückner et al. 1971; Stock 1974).

Without immediate surgical intervention following the onset of ischemia, nu-merous life-threatening complications could arise, such as hyperkalemia, he-moconcentration, and acidosis, which in turn lead to shock syndrome character-ized by decreased cardiac output, cardiac arrhythmia, and finally death due to ventricular fibrillation (Ravin et al. 1954; Eiken 1964a; van der Meer et al. 1966; Hoffmann 1969; Winninger 1973; Haimovici 1979; Prester et al. 1981; Nachbur et al. 1983). The extent of damage caused by these parameters directly correlates once again to duration of ischemia, amount of mass affected, and predominant ambient temperatures (Allen 1938; Hamel and Moe 1964; Stock et al. 1974).

The development of ischemia shock syndrome with major limb replantation can be further potentiated by peripheral factors that may add to the already exist-ing damage. Subsequent to an initially high reperfusion rate within the ischemi-cally dilated and denervated terminal vascular bed of the muscle, blood flow be-comes gradually diminished, leading to a reduced transport capacity. This imped-

Table 1. Major limb replantation: pathological conditions associated with postischemia shock syndrome

Local myopathy and capillaropathy	Multiple organ failure (MOF)
Acidosis	Systemic acidosis
Hyperosmolality	Volume deficiency
Oxygen free radicals?	Hyperkalemia
Lysosomal proteolytic enzymes	Hemoconcentration
Histamine-like mediators	Coagulation dysfunction
Coagulation dysfunction	(microembolization)
Compartment syndrome	Bacterial toxemia?

ance is directly caused by increasing edema within the limb (Stock 1974; Bondy et al. 1976; Arango et al. 1976; Matsen 1980). Progressive arterial hypotension then leads to a drop in muscle and skin perfusion, a decline in transmembrane potential, disturbance of cell volume, and diminished utilization of peripheral oxygen. Additionally, systemic hemoconcentration impairs peripheral microcirculation (Bond et al. 1967; Hagberg et al. 1970; Cunningham et al. 1971; Shires et al. 1972; Furuse et al. 1973; Sinagowitz et al. 1973; Trunkey et al. 1973; Yokoyama et al. 1979; Illner and Shires 1980; Ellsworths et al. 1981; Fontijne et al. 1985). A biochemical correlation to peripheral malperfusion has been suggested by Staples et al. (1969) and Chaudry et al. (1976). They reported finding reduced energy-rich phosphagen levels even within unaffected hind limb of rats during the end stage of hemorrhagic shock. Using the same procedure of induced tourniquet shock, however, Stock was not able to produce similar results in dogs. Amundson and Haljamäe (1976) and Jennische et al. (1979) were also unable to repeat these results in feline models.

An effect parallel to continuous drop in blood pressure is a gradual decline in arteriovenous pressure gradients within the edematous muscle compartments (Lanz 1979; Zweifach et al. 1980; Echtermeyer 1985). This further shrinkage in muscle perfusion impedes intracellular restoration during the initial postischemic phase, leading to further ischemic lesions and thus promoting disastrous interaction between the extremity and the remainder of the body. Finally, shock syndrome is also responsible for a marked anaerobic metabolism even within the unaffected limbs. This provides a clearly observable correlation between high lactate levels and death (Hofmann 1969; Karlsson et al. 1975; Amundson and Haljamäe 1976).

The above-mentioned pathophysiological cycle of factors is shown in Table 1.

2.6.2.2 Kidney Function

The first indications of a connection between postischemia syndrome and kidney dysfunction were reported just following World War I in publications describing crush/entrapment injuries (Frankenthal 1916; Hackradt 1917; Küttner 1918; Minami 1923). Hackradt observed that immediately following excavation, victims developed hematuria (*Blutharnen*) and subsequent oliguria or anuria, interpreted as acute "vasomotoric nephrosis". This same course of events was viewed by Minami as a process of "autointoxication" through acute destruction of muscle protein with methemoglobin infarction within the medulla and cortex of the kidneys.

During World War II, Bywaters (1944) studied victims of crush/entrapment injuries who had been buried during the bombings of London. He compared the histological destruction within the kidneys in these patients from "myohemoglobin" to pathological conditions within kidneys following intravasal hemolysis. An impressive loss of muscle "pigment" was also noted. Based on these findings, Bywaters formulated a recommended course of treatment for crush/entrapment patients that is still used today, including forced fluid intake, alkalization, and cooling of the extremity or, in severe cases, early amputation. In 1953, Montagnani and Simeone carried out investigations into the mechanisms of cellular liberation and systemic elimination of myoglobin in dogs subjected to 4–7.25 h of hind-limb tourniquet. Immediately following release of the tourniquet they noted impressive myoglobinemia and 10 min later, myoglobinuria. Two to four hours after restoration of limb perfusion almost normal concentration values were recorded. The same procedure was performed by Thompson et al. in 1959; however, they found serum myoglobin levels as high as 16–27 mg%, 2–4 h following tourniquet release.

It was originally thought that precipitating myoglobin within the renal tubular system was the responsible agent, as it was a common histomorphological finding in chromoprotein nephrosis. Today, experimental and clinical observations have cast some doubt on this assumption (Koslowski 1959; Weeks 1968; Haimovici 1973, 1979). It was shown by Kiessling et al. in 1981 that there is a direct quantitative connection between liberated myoglobin and rhabdomyolysis; however, clinically and experimentally no correlation has been found with the severity of renal dysfunction (Rowland et al. 1964; Haimovici 1973; Knochel 1976). This was verified by O'Regan et al. (1979) and Blachar et al. (1981) through experiments involving muscle extract infusions, which led to identical pathological changes in rats and rabbits. However, injection of a purified myoglobin preparation resulted only in an excretion of "hempigment" and proteinuria, with no decrease in the glomerular filtration fraction and no lesions of the renal tubular cells. It is no easy task to differentiate between primary renal damage caused by rhabdomyolysis and secondary lesions brought on by shock syndrome-related arterial hypotension, acidosis, and formation of microthrombi (Perri and Gorini 1952; Knochel 1976; Riede et al. 1981).

In addition to the mechanisms of destruction already discussed, there are several other possible contributors to renal shutdown, such as vasoconstriction of afferent arterioles resulting in a drop of the glomeral filtration fraction (Weeks 1968; Santangelo et al. 1982), or the influx of proteolytic lysosomal enzymes, collagen, and tissue thromboblastin with subsequent formation of microthrombi (Collan and Alho 1973; Larcan et al. 1973; Blachar et al. 1981; Riede et al. 1981; Hörl et al. 1982). Coincidently, severe systemic acidosis during shock diminishes renal excretion of myoglobin leading to precipitation in the renal tubular system (Bywaters 1944; Jasinske and Breitsch 1952; Mehl et al. 1964 b; Weeks 1968; Haimovici 1973; Biglioli et al. 1973; Winninger 1973). It therefore appears that renal failure occurring during the postischemia syndrome is multifactorally triggered.

2.6.2.3 Coagulation Disorders

Ischemic conditions within extremities cause hemostatic imbalances that, following circulatory reconstruction, can lead to functional disorders within the other organs of the body (Stallone et al. 1969; Collan and Alho 1973; Blaisdell et al. 1978; Blachar et al. 1981). Generally viewed, ischemia-induced hypercoagulability and/or hyperfibrinolysis fall into five categories.

Macroscopic Thrombus: Formation Within Major Arteries and Veins

In the presence of this condition, "milking", a Fogarty procedure, and/or irrigation are recommended clinically to precede reconstruction of a major blood vessel (Malt and McKhann 1964; Linder and Vollmar 1965; Thompson in Williams 1966; Christeas et al. 1969; Ferreira et al. 1978; Tamai et al. 1977; Johansen et al. 1982).

Erythrocyte and Thrombocyte Aggregation Formations

These can be found within the venous portion of the muscular terminal vascular bed during the initial postischemia phase (Eriksson et al. 1974, 1983). Interestingly, in rat hind-limb replantations, inverse correlations were observed between the number of venous microthrombi and limb survival (Zdeblick et al. 1985). Subsequent to long-lasting circulatory interruption, primarily focal and finally multiple venular occlusions are formed (see Sect. 2.5.4). Factors responsible for these formations are: liberation of tissue thrombokinase from ischemically damaged cells, hypoxic endothelial lesions with liberation of factor VIII and plasminogen, hindered elimination of activated coagulation products, lysosomal proteolytic enzymes, and perhaps oxygen free radicals (Letac et al. 1963; Massion and Blümel 1971; Klenermann et al. 1977; Larsson and Bergström 1978; Miller et al. 1979a, b; Gidlöf et al. 1979; Jöbsis et al. 1979; Matthias and Lasch 1981; Gerdin et al. 1985). In addition, induced capillary stenosis, postischemic edema formation, hemoconcentration, and ischemically deformed blood cells all contribute to a reduction in flow rate and to subsequent thrombus formation (see Sect. 2.5.4).

There also appears to be a correlation between thromboxane (TxA_2), prostacyclin levels, and increased platelet aggregation during tourniquet ischemia (Sullivan 1986). Blood samples obtained at time intervals up to 60 min post upper-arm cuff inflation (250 mm Hg) in human volunteers resulted in significant increases in thromboxane degradation levels as well as in notable rises in platelet aggregation.

A Flushing of Erythrocyte and Thrombocyte Aggregations, Tissue Thromboplastin, and Fibrinous Microthrombi into the Circulatory System

In cases of late embolectomy in human as well as animal subjects, autopsy investigations revealed fibrinous microthrombi within the minor pulmonary arteries, interpreted as originating from the ischemic extremities (Stallone et al. 1969; Robinson et al. 1975; Schubert et al. 1976; Blaisdell et al. 1978; Blanchar et al. 1981). Similar findings were reported by Jansson et al. (1985) in experiments in which they produced intrapulmonary aggregation of platelets and fibrinogen by standardized muscular skeletal injuries. With the postischemia syndrome it is quite difficult to decide whether coagulation disorders stem from the injured limb or are of a shock-related pulmonary origin (Riede et al. 1981; Matthias and Lasch 1981). Microembolization syndrome may also be caused by severe trauma, as maintained by Saldeen (1979) and Edfeld and Thomson (1980).

Experiments attempting to trace thrombocytes and erythrocytes within venous outflow have produced, to this point, no definitive knowledge. Following 20–120 min of tourniquet-induced ischemia within the upper-thigh region, Hirsch and Gaethgens (1965) discovered an increased level of washed-out thrombocyte aggregates in blood samples taken from the femoral vein and the vena cava employing a pressure-filtration system (*Siebungsdruckverfahren*). Using photoelectric methods, Lauterjung and Stock (1973) were able to differentiate between aggregate formations in the femoral vein and in the vena cava following 5 h of hind-limb tourniquet in dogs. Despite a rapid increase in the number of aggregates within the efflux of the femoral vein during the early reperfusion phase, parallel blood samples collected from the vena cava gave no evidence of aggregation formation. They therefore assumed that disaggregation mechanisms within circulating blood hindered the influx of aggregates into the pulmonary vascular bed. Further results were reported by Siebert et al. (1975 a, b) from experiments involving a 3-h hind-limb tourniquet in dogs. Using an agglometer they were able to observe maximal aggregate formations 10 min after reperfusion to the limb. One hour later, however, normal levels were found. Despite significant drops in thrombocyte counts and fibrinogen levels within systemic blood, only a few of the animals actually developed fibrin and thrombocyte thrombi within the pulmonary vascular bed.

Increase in Fibrinolytic Activity

Further ischemia-induced changes within the coagulation system of human subjects were observed by Larsson et al. (1981) during 1–3 h of upper-arm tourniquet with exsanguination. Biopsies on skin and superficial veins performed during this interval revealed a clear increase in fibrinolytic activity (histochemical method according to Todd). Four to six days later, however, normalization took place. A systemic increase in fibrinolytic activity 15 min after reinitiation of perfusion was observed by Klenermann et al. (1977).

These alterations observed in orthopedic patients took place in the arms and legs 15 min after a 50-min tourniquet period. During the procedure thrombocyte and fibrinogen levels remained stable.

Drops in Fibrinogen, Antithrombin III, and Plasminogen; Rise in Fibrin-split Products and Fibrin Peptide A

Further information pertaining to the systemic tolerance level of the coagulation system following ischemic insult was offered by Miller et al. (1979 b), gathered from studies carried out with large primates. After release of a 2.5-h upper-arm tourniquet, significant drops in fibrinogen, antithrombin III, and plasminogen levels within plasma, concomitant with a rise in fibrin-split products and fibrin peptide A were observed. Five to thirty minutes following reperfusion, however, laboratory parameters indicative of initiating coagulation and fibrinolysis returned to normal.

2.6.2.4 Toxemia and Infection

It has been more than a half century since medical scientists began trying to understand the pathophysiological mechanisms involved in the dramatic decreases in circulatory parameters and organ failure connected with postischemia syndrome. In experiments it was demonstrated that massage of the extremities exacerbated the symptoms (Cannon and Bayliss 1919; Bayliss 1919). Plasma drawn from such ischemically insulted extremities and injected into a healthy subject produced the onset of circulatory depression. The result of these studies was the assumption that toxic-related substances were involved (Aub 1944; Aub et al. 1945; Perestoronin in Lapchinski 1960; LeTac et al. 1963). In the search for a causative substance, Dyckerhoff (Dyckerhoff and Schörcher 1938–39; Dyckerhoff et al. 1938–39) prepared specimens of muscle pulp, from which he was convinced to have isolated a specific myotoxin, „Frühgift". His experimental results, however, were more than likely attributable to bacterial toxins. Bollman and Flock (1944) showed that ATP and its degradation products could be ruled out as factors causing toxicity development, while in 1952, Green and Stoner published reports claiming nucleotide fragments, together with thromboplastin, fat, and magnesium, to be the elements responsible. Yet another point of view was offered by Zamecnik et al. (1945), who stated that a protein existing within ischemic muscle exsudate was the agent causing toxicity. Interestingly enough, as early as 1930, Blalock, and in 1945 Kety et al., postulated the theory that plasma loss into an ischemically damaged extremity is a pathogenetic mechanism sufficient to lead to shock syndrome, but that this could actually be reversed through full blood transfusions. Injection of centrifuged muscle extract taken from an ischemically damaged limb or serum from an end-stage postischemia shock-syndrome study animal failed to produce circulatory breakdown in heparinized controls (Roone and Wilson 1935; Mehl et al. 1964b; Eiken et al. 1964). These results support the previously mentioned findings of Blalock (1930). The possibility that toxic products might exit from the ischemic limb via the lymphatic channels was also looked into by Katzenstein et al. (1943). Injection of collected lymph, however, following tourniquet release, did not produce evidence for development of shock syndrome. A further factor perhaps responsible for false-positive experimental results was the rapid bacterial contamination of the muscle exudate. In autopsies on victims of postischemia shock syndrome, *Clostridium perfringens* and *Clostridium oedematiens, Escherichia coli,* and anaerobic bacteria were found, owing to the fact that ischemic muscle provides a perfect culture (Wilson and Roome 1936; Aub 1944; Nathanson et al. 1945; Pope et al. 1945).

The body's endogenous defense mechanisms against infection are significantly weakened through the development of ischemia within an extremity and subsequent shock syndrome. Peripheral oxygen deficiencies are correlated with a decline in oxidation mechanisms necessary for bacterial destruction carried out by macrophages (Babior 1978; Weissman et al. 1979). Reduced hemoglobin causes a marked slowdown in polymorphonuclear leukocyte activity against *E. coli* and *Staphylococcus aureus* (Welch et al. 1982). Finally, shock syndrome itself is associated with sluggish phagocytosis of leukocytes (Burkhardt and Stankovic 1973).

Similar conditions can be observed in human major limb replantation involving extremities with crush injuries along the stump site and/or severed portion, or in cases of distended normothermic ischemia resulting in extensive edema formation. In these instances, septic toxic reactions are most feared, and should they occur, only urgent reamputation can prevent the possibility of death (Denotter 1968; Frank 1972; Chishueit 1975; Sixth People's Hospital Shanghai 1975; Ferreira et al. 1978; Maurer et al. 1979, 1985; Berger 1983). Contradicting the theory of bacteria-induced toxemia in the development of postischemia shock syndrome, there have been clinical observations, as in cases of late embolectomy, in which severe shock syndrome developed in the absence of traumatic soft tissue injury or bacterial contamination (Haimovici 1979).

3 Materials and Methods

In the past, the aim of the vast majority of perfusion and storage methods was to hinder the advancing onset of muscle cell and capillary bed injury as well as to block the development of postischemia syndrome. It should be noted, however, that all experimental and clinical aspects of such therapy have no significant impact if during the ischemic interval, the reperfusion phase, or the rehabilitation period one or more of the following criteria are not met:

1. Protection of skeletal muscles through synthesis of energy-rich phosphagens
2. Washout of acidic metabolites, potassium, cellular degradation products, and cellular mediators to obstruct the "reperfusion effect" and clotting disorders
3. Good rheological access to the ischemically stenosed capillary vascular bed
4. No significant injury to the remainder of the body as a whole
5. Technically uncomplicated execution of the perfusion procedure
6. Inclusion of postoperative regeneration phase

Animal experiments should therefore provide substantial evidence for the cytoprotective effect and should avoid early and late complications with post ischemia syndrome.

3.1 Product Description

The oxygenated, stroma-free hemoglobin (HbPP) solution employed (Bonhard 1976) was obtained from erythrocytes separated from outdated human whole blood. Following chemical sterilization and hemolysis, the stroma lipids were separated. An improvement in the oxygen binding curve was achieved by replacing the natural 2.3 DPG (diphosphoglycerate) with the vitamin-B derivative pyridoxal phosphate. The solution entailed no species specificity and no ABO incompatibility and had a pH of 7.4. With the corpuscular components removed, the solution possessed excellent rheological properties: relative kinematical viscosity of 1.3 with a mean molecular weight of 65000. Further physiological and biochemical properties were:

– p 50 value with pH 7.4 at 37° C. 27–30 mm Hg
– Colloidal osmotic pressure – 30 mm Hg
– Osmolality of the 6% solution – 280 mosmol

Electrolytes

Na^+ 145   mmol K^+ 3.2 mmol

Ca^{++}	1.5 mmol	Mg^{++}	1.1 mmol
Cl^-	100 mmol	HCO_3^-	20.0 mmol
SO_4^{--}	1.0 mmol		

Thrombogenic and allergenic characteristics have so far not been observed.

With temperature maintained between 2° and 8° C, stability of the solution could be insured for up to 8 months in glass bottles.

At the onset of the experiment series, oxygenation by means of aeration with carbogen was performed in a magnetic stirring system immediately prior to initiation of perfusion. Further along into the series, a previously oxygenated hemoglobin solution (which can also be safely stored for up to 8 months at a temperature of 2°–8° C and constant pO_2 was provided by Biotest Institute, Frankfurt, West Germany. Perfusion of the rat hind limbs was performed using the original solution; for canine hind-limb perfusion the already oxygenated hemoglobin preparation was employed.[1]

3.2 Analytic Methods

3.2.1 Storage and Perfusion in Isolated Rat Hind Limbs

Male Sprague-Dawley rats of the same age and weighing 400–450 g were used. All of the animals were housed individually and maintained under identical living conditions, which included day/night light regulation, controlled temperature, special diet (Altromin 1324), and water intake ad libitum.

In order to avoid circadian rhythm interference, the experiments were routinely started between 8:00 and 9:00 a.m.

Following a short exposure to ether, the animals were killed (neck break) and careful preparation of the femoral vein and artery within the thigh region (23 ± 1.4 g) was carried out. Skin from the extremity was removed at the point of the ankle plane, leaving the fascial compartments intact.

Preliminary experiments were conducted in an effort to clarify whether perfusion with an oxygenated hemoglobin solution had any direct influence on energy-rich phosphate production. There was evidence of a protective effect on the skeletal musculature with orthograde perfusion of an oxygenated hemoglobin preparation. All other randomly attempted methods such as perfusion with physically oxygenized Ringer's lactate solution, retrograde perfusion with an oxygenated HbPP solution, and orthograde perfusion with a non-oxygenated hemoglobin solution produced clearly inferior morphological and biochemical results.

---

[1] Hemoglobin solutions are tested and/or produced by:

1. B. Braun Melsungen AG (correspondence: H. Feller, M. D.), 3508 Melsungen, West Germany
2. Intermedicat GmbH, 45 Gerliswil Street, 6020 Emmenbrücke, Switzerland
3. Ajinomoto Inc., 5–8 Kyobashi 1-chome, Chuo-ku, Chiyoda-ku 104, Tokyo, Japan
4. Fisons plc., Fison House, Princess Street, Ipswich, Suffolk I91 1QH, Great Britain
5. Laboratoire d'Hématologie et Physiologie, Faculté des Sciences Pharm. et Biol., Bp 403, 54001, Nancy, Cedex, France
6. Statko Inc. (correspondence: F. de Venuto, M. D.), Petaluma, Los Angeles, CA, USA

Thereafter, the standard clinically recommended process of preservation (cold storage of the limb at 4° C) was tested for its superiority over those results obtained from orthograde perfusion with an oxygenated HbPP solution. Twenty-four hind-limb preparations were randomized and subsequently assigned to one of the following treatment protocols:

1. Following initial ischemia for 2 h at 22° C (muscle tissue sample collection at 0, 1, and 2 h) and storage at 4° C for 4 h (collection at 3, 5, and 6 h), the preparations were wrapped (according to surgical replantation routine) with a sterile compress and sealed with waterproof packing in a plastic pouch. The watertight pouch was then submerged into an ice bath in order to maintain a central temperature of 4° C.
2. Following initial ischemia for 2 h at 22° C (muscle tissue sample collection at 0, 1, and 2 h), perfusion was initiated with an oxygenated hemoglobin solution for 4 h (collection at 3, 5, and 6 h). Perfusion was performed through cannulation of the femoral artery with a polyethylene catheter (0.8 mm in diameter, 10 cm long) which was positioned at the branch of the deep femoral artery and secured with a 6-0 silk ligature. A roller pump system (Watson-Marlow Pump Type MHRE 22) ensured constant flow rate of 5 ml/100 g tissue/min to the wellsecured amputated limb. A longitudinal incision of the femoral vein provided unhampered outflow from the venous system.

Oxygenation of the hemoglobin solution was achieved through aeration with carbogen within a magnetic stirring system. Experimental levels were pO_2 146.21 ± 29.48 Torr and pCO_2 35.56 ± 8.47 Torr ($n = 6$, $X \pm SX$). In contrast to the first group ("dry-cooling" at 4° C) it was possible to maintain a constant temperature of 22° C throughout the entire perfusion procedure.

As a parameter for muscular metabolism, the intracellular energy-rich phosphagens ATP (adenosine triphosphate), CP (creatine phosphate), and lactate were examined using enzyme optical test methods according to Warburg (1948).

With a liquid nitrogen-cooled steel puncture needle (Travenol Tru-cut), standard muscle tissue samples were harvested from the proximal third of the anterior tibial compartment (Wollenberger et al. 1960). Core biopsies with wet tissue weights of 4–11 mg were collected at 0, 1, and 2 h during ischemia as well as at 3, 5 and 6 h during the other different treatment methods.

Following immediate submersion into liquid nitrogen, the samples were prepared for evaluation according to the techniques of Bergmeyer (1962). Tissue samples combined with an ice-cold solution of 3.5% percloric acid (w/v) were subjected to blade homogenization (Ultra Turrax, Kunkel, Stauffen) at maximal rpm, and specimen weight was thereafter determined using a microbalance. Through centrifugation at 16 000 g in an ultraperformance centrifuge (WKF, Type G, 50K) at 0° C, the acid-insoluble components were separated, and subsequent to the addition of potassium bicarbonate, the acid-soluble supernatant was adjusted to a pH of 6.0. Potassium salts that had precipitated from the percloric acid portion were filtered out and the supernatant was introduced to the chemical test preparation. Absorption was determined in an Eppendorf photometer using temperature-controlled, flow-through curvette cells and wave lengths prescribed by Bergmeyer (1962).

3.2.2 Analysis of Perfusate

Gas Analysis. During the perfusion process in group 2, samples of outflowing venous perfusate were collected at 15 min and 1, 2, 3, and 4 h from heparinized capillary sites (D 551/12.5) for subsequent gas analysis utilizing a radiometer (Copenhagen BMS, 3MK 2).

Potassium. At 10, 15, and 30 min and 1, 2, 3, and 4 h, samples were collected in order to determine potassium concentration levels (radiometer, Copenhagen KNA 1 Na-K Analyzer, and Instrumentation Laboratories Flame Photometer 743, half-automated evaluations).

Electron-Optical Examination. At completion of the perfusion procedure, cubic muscle samples were harvested from the cranial portion of the tibial compartment and prepared for electron-optical examination. The 0.5 mm × 1 mm × 2 mm cubic samples were fixed in a phosphate-buffered 2.5% glutaraldehyde solution (pH 7.2), and this was followed by counter fixation with osmium tetroxide. Embedding was carried out in an acsending acetone series in Vestopal. The microtomed sections were counterstained with lead citrate and uranyl acetate. The magnifications presented within the figures are actual representation provided by the electron microscope employed.

3.2.3 Storage and Perfusion in Canine Hind Limbs

A total of 38 mixed-breed dogs with an average body weight of 17 ± 2 kg were used as test subjects. The dogs were quarantined for 4 weeks prior to usage, during which time they were dewormed and vaccinated against any common infectious disease. All animals were housed individually and maintained on a standard diet, with feeding times limited to 1 h and water intake ad libitum.

In order to avoid possible circadian rhythm interference, all daily experimental procedures were begun on a regular schedule between the hours of 8:00 a.m. and 8:00 p.m.

Preliminary surgery was carried out in 13 dogs to test the complicated surgical technique, the life-supporting perioperative therapy, and postoperative management. The following protocol was found to be successful in creating a defined muscle ischemia without permanent concurrent damage to the remainder of the body.

Anesthesia and Infusion Therapy. Following sedation with 0.05 ml/kg body wt. Combelene (i.m.), the animals tolerated induction of inhalation narcosis (2.5 vol% halothane and N_2O/Oxygen 5:2) administered through an animal mask. Endotracheal intubation was carried out using a 32-Charrier Rüsch intubation tube. Care was taken to ensure that both lungs were fully ventilated. Upon completion of anesthesia induction, halothane administration was reduced to 1.5 vol%. In order to avoid the possibility of regionally insufficient ventilation during the course of the procedure, the animals were periodically repositioned and closely observed. Throughout the 10-h procedure the dogs breathed spontaneously and received a standardized fluid load via a Braunule 1.2-mm cannula according to the following schedule:

1. Up to the end of the third procedural hour, the dog received a total of 40 ml Ringer's solution/kg body wt. with 0.5 mEq NA HCO_3/kg body wt.
2. Two hours following rejoining of the extremity to the autogenous circulation, administration of a total of 40 ml Ringer's solution/kg body wt. with 0.5 mval NA HCO_3/kg body wt. was repeated.
3. Prior to reversal of anesthesiy, an infusion of 5.5% colloidal solution from oxypolygelatine (Gelifundol, 20 ml/kg body wt.) was administered.

Determination of blood pressure and collection of arterial blood samples were accomplished through cannulation of the left femoral artery and placement of a Vygon catheter (7.5 cm, 1.5×2.00 mm) at the aortic bifurcation. Following fixation and subcutaneous tunneling, the catheter was connected to a Statham Pressure Transducer (Hato Rey 6781, P23 IA) via an interpositioned Vygon Lectro catheter (nos. 115 and 20, 200 cm, 0.5 mm).

Continuous systolic and diastolic blood pressures were recorded on a four-channel printer (Simonson and Weck Pso 21/MVD with pressure amplifier) with simultaneous control of mean arterial pressure. In parallel, the pulse rate and ECG were registered via pin electrodes attached to the skin surface of the extremity.

Preparation for the actual procedure was then undertaken. The right hind limbs were shaved, sterilized three times with Dijozol, and draped. Throughout the surgical procedure rectal temperatures were recorded and the animals were kept at an average body temperature of $35°$–$36°$ C with the aid of a heat lamp and blanket.

Circumferential incision of the skin and adjacent soft tissues in the region of the mid thigh was followed by concentric muscle dissection at the subtrochanteric level. To guarantee postoperative extension within the knee joint, the ventral belly of the thigh extender was freed just above the patella. All other muscle groups were incised step by step using a thermocautery, whereby a number of the major vessels were ligated (3-0 Dexon). The femoral and ischiatic nerves and the femoral artery and vein were left carefully intact. The nutrient vessels of the nerves were microcoagulated over a length of 8 cm at the level of the amputation.

Osteotomy of the femur at its midpoint using an oscillating saw was undertaken and a 1-cm segment was resected. A functionally stable osteosynthesis was performed through a 4-bore, $1/2$ tubular or 6-bore, $1/3$ tubular plate, according to the prescribed method of the Osteosynthesis Association (AO International). Interfragmental compression was placed on the osteosynthesis through eccentric drilling of the screw holes. The various muscles were adapted using single stitches of Vicryl 1-0, and the thigh extender was fixed onto the patella. Thereafter, the skin was closed with vertical mattress sutures (nylon 3-0), leaving free access to the vessels.

Since at this point the extremities were perfused exclusively by the femoral artery and vein, complete ischemia could be achieved by clamping the two vessels with bulldog clamps at the level of the inguinal ligament. To observe the existence of total ischemia following clamping, the femoral vein was incised for a short

Table 2. Experimental protocols for three groups

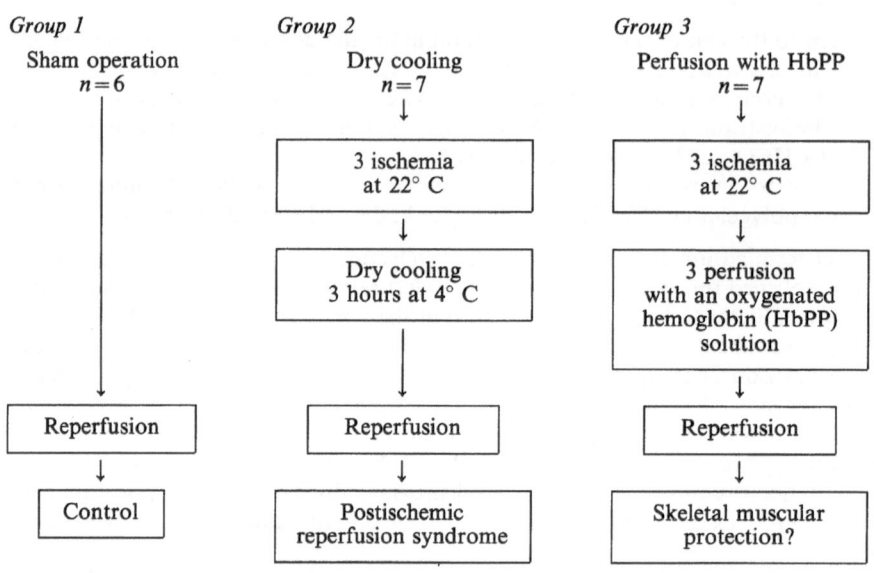

length distal to the bulldog clamp. This incision also provided for free outflow of the perfusate and it was closed at the end of the procedure with a continuous suture (6-0 nylon).

The effect of extremity perfusion with an oxygenated HbPP solution on the reperfusion phase and the morphological alterations within the musculature following the ischemic interval were determined with the animals randomly assigned to three groups (Table 2).

Group 1 – Sham Operations (n=6). In this group a neurovascular pedicle graft of the hind limb was prepared and the vessels were clamped for 5 min (intimal lesion). The femoral vein was incised and subsequently closed with a continuous suture (6-0 nylon). Following reconstruction of the dissected structures, the animals were kept under narcosis for 10 h.

Group 2 – Cold Storage (n=7). A neurovascular pedicle graft of the hind limb was prepared. The femoral vessels were clamped for 3 h, resulting in ischemia at 22° C. Subsequently, the extremities were packed in compresses, placed in a watertight plastic pouch, and submerged in an ice bath for 3 h. This procedure resulted in a temperature drop to 4° C within the extremity, as is the case in common clinical practice. Following a total of 6 h ischemia (3 h at 22° C and 3 h in cold storage at 4° C), the femoral vein was sutured and the clamps removed. The skin over the inguinal region was subsequently closed using the Donati suture technique and 3-0 nylon.

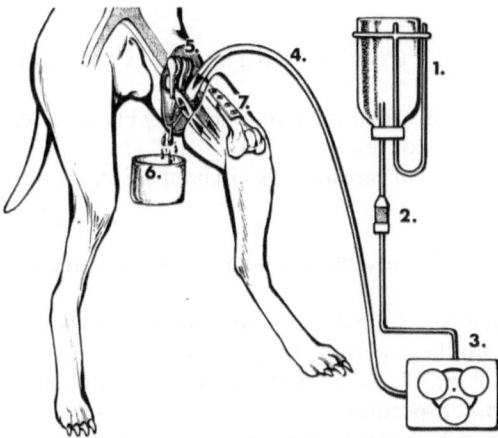

Fig. 2. Perfusion to a vessel pedicle graft during the ischemic interval. *1*, Oxygenated hemoglobin solution; *2*, special filter in the infusion tube; *3*, roller pump; *4*, catheterization of femoral artery; *5*, proximal clamping of femoral vein and artery; *6*, venous efflux; *7*, functionally stable osteosynthesis after resection of femur segment

Group 3 – Perfusion with an Oxygenated HbPP Solution (n=7). A neurovascular pedicle graft of the hind limb was prepared, as in the other two groups. Following 3 h of ischemia at 22° C, achieved by clamping off the vessels, a 3-h perfusion of the isolated extremity was performed using a previously oxygenated and stored hemoglobin solution. The bottles containing HbPP were punctured and the contents allowed to flow foam free into the perfusion system through a filtration system (Biotest Institute). The system was connected to a plastic catheter (Vygon 75 cm, 1.5×2 mm) which was placed into the side branch of the femoral artery and advanced up to the bifurcation of the deep femoral artery. The cather was fixed to the adductor musculature using 3-0 Dexon suture.

Perfusion was performed using a roller pump system (Watson Marlow MHRE 22) with adjustable flow rates. The venous backflow was collected as it exited from the incised femoral vein. Figure 2 illustrates this technically simple setup. Following the initial 3-h ischemic phase, a perfusion flow rate of 2 ml/100 g tissue/min was chosen for the initial 10 min and this was subsequently increased to 4 ml/100 g tissue/min. Shortly before reestablishment of autogenous circulation to the hind limb, the limb was flushed with 200 ml Ringer's solution with gravity perfusion until the venous efflux appeared pale red.

Postoperatively, the animals in all three groups were caged individually and maintained on a balanced, standardized canine diet with the addition of defined portions of canned dog food and water consumption ad libitum. Tetracycline and ampicillin (1.5 g/day) were administered for 5 days postoperatively.

3.2.4 Determination of Reperfusion Effect

In all three experimental groups, the following blood collection and measurement intervals were chosen for determination of the reperfusion effect (declamping phenomenon):

- pH of aortic blood
1. Before release of the femoral vein and artery clamps, 6 h into the experimental procedure
2. Fifteen minutes following release of the femoral vein and artery clamps, i.e., 6 h, 15 min into the experimental procedure
3. One hour following release of the femoral vein and artery clamps, i.e., 7 h into the experimental procedure
- Mean arterial pressure
1. Before release of the femoral vein and artery clamps, 6 h into the experimental procedure
2. Five and 15 minutes following release of the femoral vein and artery clamps, i.e., 6 h, 5 min and 6 h, 15 min into the experimental procedure
3. One and two hours following release of the femoral vein and artery clamps, i.e., 7 and 8 h into the experimental procedure

In addition, pCO_2, pO_2, HCO_3, and base excess levels were recorded in arterial blood samples at varying times (6 h, 15 min, and 7 h); these data may provide a basis for further hypotheses in future experiments. The concentrations of inorganic phosphate (Pi) at 6 (0), 7 (1), and 8 h (2 h reperfusion) were also systemmatically determined.

For blood gas analysis, aortic blood samples were drawn from the femoral artery catheter, placed into heparinized capillaries (D 551-12.5), and analyzed in a Copenhagen Radiometer.

Using the same method the washout effect within the hind limbs was determined; hemoglobin perfusate was collected from the venous efflux at 5, 15, 30, 60, 120, and 180 min following the initiation of perfusion. As parameters, pH, pO_2, pCO_2, HCO_3, and base excess levels were measured.

Determination of the arterial Pi concentration levels was performed following the collection of 5-ml blood samples from the femoral artery. One milliliter was discarded and the remainder of the samples subjected to centrifugation at 3000 rpm; it was then analyzed using a photometric redox reaction.

3.2.5 Histological and Electron-Optical Analyses

Muscle samples from the proximal third of the anterior tibial muscle and the medial head of the gastrocnemius of both the operated and contralateral limbs were collected at 24 and 48 h, 5, 6, and 8 days, 3 months, and at 1 and 1.5 years postoperatively, in order to assess the morphological and ultrastructural postoperative course.

With the animal under brief anesthesia, (0.3 ml/kg Polamivet and 0.02 ml/kg Combelene) the compartment fascia was opened over a length of 8 cm. Muscle samples were harvested by isometric placement on a cork board. Specimens of 0.5, 1, and 2×0.05 cm were cut and subsequently fixed for 8 h in a 4% formalin phosphate-buffered solution (pH 7.2). Embedding was done in paraffin (Paraplast Plus) using an ascending alcohol series. Microtome slices of 3 μm were stained with H and E and PAS using standardized techniques (Romeis 1968). Connective tissue was identified using van Gieson's technique.

In parallel to the histological specimens, muscle blocks ($0.5 \times 1 \times 2$ mm) were excised for electron-optical analysis using the same technique as was employed with the rat skeletal musculature. Following removal of the muscle samples, the compartments were carefully closed with continuous suturing of the fascia (3-0 Dexon) once hemostasis had been secured with thermocautery. The skin was closed using Donati stitches (3-0 nylon). The same technique was employed to collect muscle tissue samples from the contralateral unoperated limbs, which were used as controls.

At 24 and 48 h, 3 months, and 1 and 1.5 years postoperatively, tissue samples were taken from the liver and kidneys for the purpose of histological examination. The samples were fixed for 8 h in a 4% phosphate-buffered formalin solution and subsequently embedded in paraffin. Cuts of 3 μm were obtained with a microtome blade and the tissues were subsequently stained with H and E and PAS according to Romeis (1968). Iron traces were identified using the Berlin-blue reaction, while hemoglobin was located utilizing the staining technique of Okajima.

3.2.6 Washout Effect and Quantitative Determination of Residua

Since it was assumed that in the presence of preexisting ischemic damage to the muscle capillary bed, the stroma-free hemoglobin solution employed passed over into the interstitial space during long-term perfusion, it was deemed necessary to determine residua mass. These investigations were performed in the radioisotope laboratory of the Biotest Serum Institute, Offenbach, Federal Republic of Germany. The coupling of hemoglobin molecules with iodine 125 produced a test substance with an activity of 8571 ± 340 cpm/0.1 ml ($n = 5$).

3.2.7 Method of Perfusion

Following subtrochanteric amputation of the hind limb in five mixed-breed dogs, Vygon catheters (1.5×2.75 cm) were placed into the femoral arteries; the preparations were then fixed to a stand positioned over a collection funnel. During the procedure all perfusate exiting from the venous circulation drained directly from the funnel into a sterilized decontamination flask.

After the initial ischemic phase at $22°$ C, a 3-h perfusion procedure employing a radiolabeled and oxygenated hemoglobin solution was carried out (flow rate: 4 ml ^{125}I-labeled HbPP/100 g tissue/min). Then, using a nonlabeled hemoglobin solution, the perfusion was continued for 1 h (flow rate same as above), and samples were collected from the venous exit site at 5, 10, 15, 20, 25, 30, 40, 45, and 60 min. With a gamma counter (Gamma-Counter Packard, Type 5 120), a descending curve was constructed.

Subsequent to perfusion of the extremities with the radiolabeled HbPP solution, as well as at the conclusion of the experiments, tissue samples were taken from the skin, subcutaneous tissue, the anterior tibial muscle, and the gastrocnemius muscle with the intent of performing residual mass studies using the method previously described.

3.3 Statistical Methods[2]

Univariate analysis of variance (ANOVA) for repeated measures was found to be a suitable method for comparing two or more samples with repeated measurements on the same subject. Differences between the samples and variations over a time could be tested simultaneously within these models.

Inductive statistical analysis was performed for the following most relevant parameters: ATP, CP, lactate, pH value, mean blood pressure, and pulse rate. The corresponding values for ATP, CP, and lactate, measured 2 h following ischemia at 22° C, were used as covariates for the respective evaluations performed later, following perfusion with an oxygenated HbPP solution and dry cooling. Mean blood pressure, pulse rate, and pH value were compared after storage for 3 h at 22° C, dry cooling at 4° C, perfusion with an HbPP solution, or no treatment (replantation without ischemia).

Two-factor ANOVA with repeated measurements on the factor time (room temperature 22° C) was found to be an appropriate model for evaluating the accumulated data. In order to conform to the prerequisites of the ANOVA model, it was necessary to transform the data to normal scores. The significance level was assumed to be 5%.

All other controls were evaluated by descriptive methods only, with the intent of using these data in future studies. They were described by arithmetical means and correspond to standard deviations.

---

[2] Experimental and statistical analyses were performed by the Institute for Numerical Statistics, Cologne, Federal Republic of Germany.

4 Results

4.1 Storage and Reperfusion Attempts

4.1.1 Metabolic Studies

Comparison of the clinically recommended technique of dry cooling at 4° C vs. perfusion with an oxygenated HbPP solution was initially performed by determining the intracellular levels of the energy-rich phosphagens ATP and CP as well as the intracellular lactate concentrations within isolated rat hind limbs. Tissue samples were harvested using a stop-freeze technique at 0, 1, and 2 h at a room temperature of 22° C and at 3, 5, and 6 h of treatment. Twenty-four amputated limbs were randomized and each probed three times for evaluation. The results are presented in Figs. 3–5.

In the case of all three parameters (ATP, CP, and lactate), a significant difference was found between the treatment protocols and the change over time ($P < 0.01$; Table 3).

4.1.2 Experiments with Perfusates

In order to evaluate the washout effect during the perfusion process, standardized samples of venous perfusate were collected at 10 and 15 min and at 1, 2 ($n = 2$), 3, and 4 h from a total of six hind limbs. The samples were then analyzed for potassium levels.

The mean values are depicted in Fig. 6. Following an initially high concentration of 10.8 mEq/l, the potassium levels within the perfusate sank to 8.7 mval/l

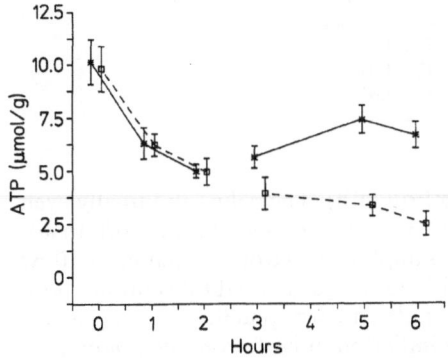

Fig. 3. ATP concentrations within the anterior tibial muscle of the rat following 2 h of ischemia at 22° C. (——•——), 4 h HbPP perfusion ($n = 6$); (--□--), 4 h dry cooling at 4° C ($n = 6$)

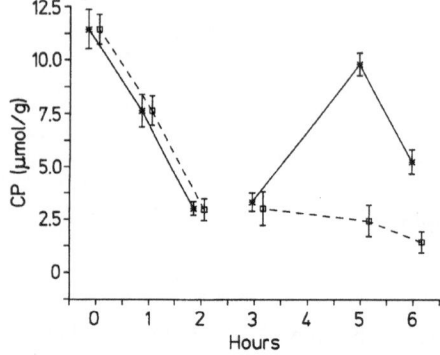

Fig. 4. Creatine phosphate concentrations within the anterior tibial muscle of the rat following 2 h of ischemia at 22° C. (—*—), 4 h HbPP perfusion ($n=6$); (−−□−−), 4 h dry cooling at 4° C ($n=6$)

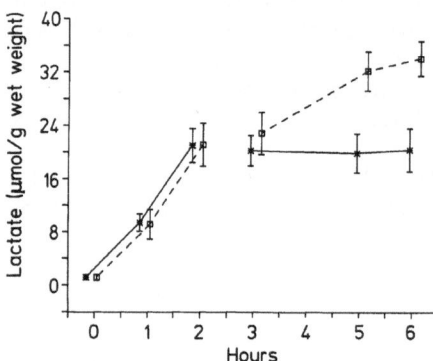

Fig. 5. Lactate levels within the anterior tibial muscle of the rat following 2 h of ischemia at 22° C. (—*—), 4 h HbPP perfusion ($n=6$); (−−□−−), 4 h dry cooling at 4° C ($n=6$)

Table 3. Results of analysis of variance of parameters of muscle cell metabolism following normal range transformation of values (covariable value after 2 h)

Parameter	Difference/ treatment methods	Difference/time
ATP	$P < 0.01$	$P < 0.01$
CP	$P < 0.01$	$P < 0.01$
Lactate	$P < 0.01$	$P < 0.01$

(15 min), 8.37 mEq/l (30 min) and 6.49 mEq/l (1 h). The values did finally even off, and were at 2 h 7.13 mEq/l, at 3 h 6.61 mEq/l, and at 4 h 6.74 mEq/l. In addition, pO_2 and pCO_2 were determined in samples taken from the venous outflow ($n=6$; Fig. 7). In the case of perfusion with an oxygenated HbPP solution, both parameters showed an intersecting curve pattern corresponding to the primary acidosis. Fifteen minutes later, following initiation of perfusion, the *venous* pO_2 mean value was 55.0 mm Hg with a pCO_2 of 83.5 mm Hg; the pO_2 then rapidly rose to 83.9 mm Hg, while the pCO_2 decreased to 42.6 mm Hg.

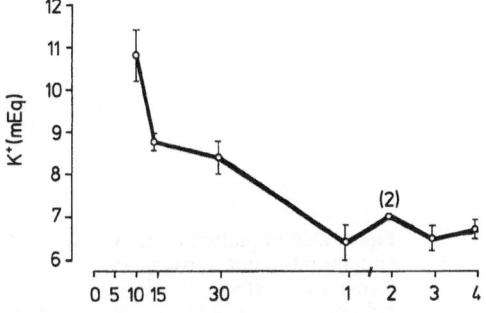

Fig. 6. Potassium concentrations within venous efflux following 2 h of ischemia at 22° C and subsequent 4-h perfusion with an oxygenated HbPP solution in rat hind limbs ($n=6$)

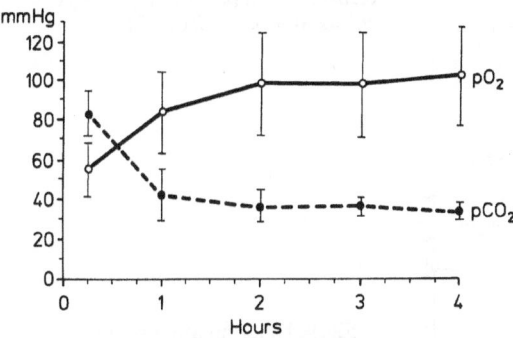

Fig. 7. pO_2 and pCO_2 in venous efflux following 2 h of ischemia at 22° C and subsequent 4-h perfusion with an oxygenated HbPP solution in rat hind limbs ($n=6$)

Following 2 h of perfusion, the pO_2 reached a mean value of 98.1 mm Hg with a corresponding decrease in pCO_2 to 35.8 mm Hg. At 3 and 4 h of perfusion the pO_2 and pCO_2 values remained stable.

4.1.3 Systemic Measurements, Reperfusion Effect

To investigate the influence of HbPP perfusion on the magnitude of the reperfusion effect, 20 dogs were randomly assigned to one of the three experimental groups. Following an ischemic period of 3 h at 22° C, the hind limbs in the hypothermic storage group were maintained at 4° C for another 3-h period ($n=7$). In the second group, a 3-h perfusion procedure employing an oxygenated HbPP solution followed ($n=7$). To eliminate potential sources of error resulting from the considerable amputation trauma as well as from the prolonged anesthesia, a group of sham experiments were deemed necessary ($n=6$).

During the initial 3-h ischemic phase and the subsequent various treatments of the neurovascular pedicled extremities, neither the circulatory parameters nor the arterial pH values exhibited relevant alterations under identical anesthesia and infusion programs.

As a measure of the reperfusion effect, the pH within arterial circulation was evaluated immediately before restoration of blood flow to the extremity (i.e., at 6 h as well as at 15 min (6 h, 15 min) and 1 h into reperfusion (7 h).

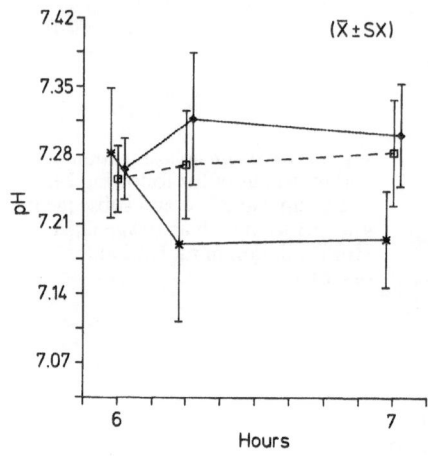

Fig. 8. Determination of pH within circulating canine aortic blood. Reperfusion effect following 3-h ischemia at 22° C and: (———■———) sham procedure ($n = 6$); (——□——) HbPP perfusion – *3 h* ($n = 7$); or (——*——) dry cooling at 4° C – *3 h* ($n = 7$)

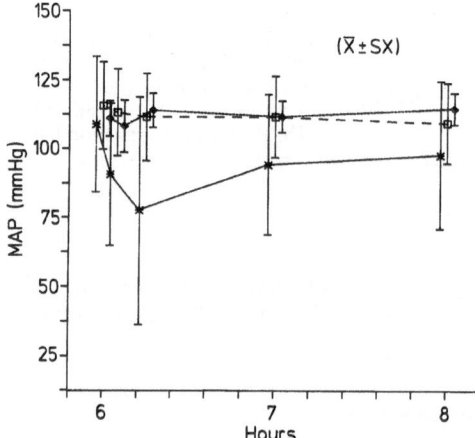

Fig. 9. Determination of mean arterial pressure (MAP) within canine aorta. Reperfusion effect following 3 h of ischemia at 22° C and: (———■———) sham procedure ($n = 5$); (——□——) HbPP perfusion – *3 h* ($n = 6$); or (——*——) dry cooling at 4° C – *3 h* ($n = 7$)

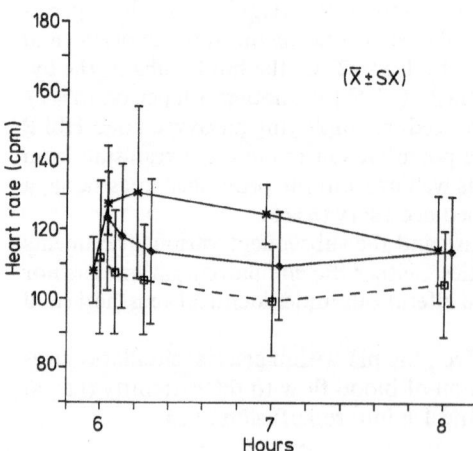

Fig. 10. Determination of heart rate/min. Reperfusion effect following 3 h of ischemia at 22° C and: (———■———) sham procedure ($n = 5$); (——□——) HbPP perfusion – *3 h* ($n = 6$); (——*——) dry cooling at 4° C – *3 h* ($n = 7$)

Parallel to this, the mean arterial pressure (MAP) and the heart rate (HR) were registered at 6 h (before restoration of blood flow) as well as at 5 and 15 min and 1 and 2 h following reperfusion (6 h 5 min, 6 h 15 min, 7 h, and 8 h respectively). Due to a defect within the apparatus, one animal in the reperfusion group and one from the sham-experiment group were left out of the MAP and HR results. Figures 8, 9 and 10 demonstrate these parameters as mean values ± SD. With $P < 0.05$ as the level of significance, the pH and HR exhibited significant differences at $P < 0.01$ and the MAP at $P < 0.05$ when treatment regimes were compared (Table 4).

Table 4. Parameters of reperfusion effect (declamping phenomenon) in dogs. Result of analysis of variance following normal range transformation of variables

Parameter	Difference/ treatment methods	Difference/time
pH	$P < 0.01$	$P < 0.01$
Mean arterial pressure	$P < 0.05$*	$P < 0.01$
Heart frequency	$P < 0.01$	$P < 0.01$

* Not significant.

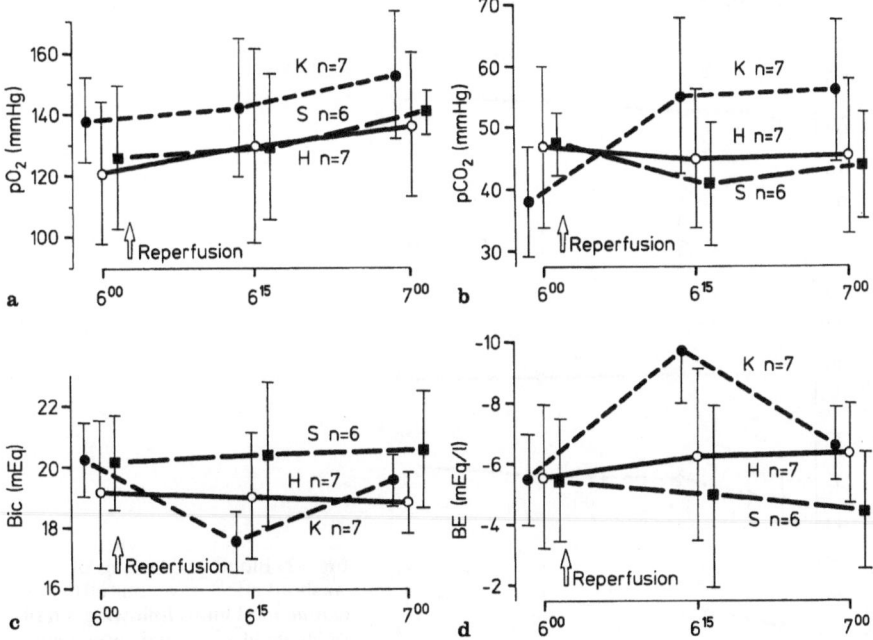

Fig. 11 a–d. Gas analysis in circulating aortic canine blood – **a** pO_2, **b** pCO_2, **c** bicarbonate, **d** base excess. Reperfusion effect following 3 h of ischemia at 22° C and: (---●---) dry cooling at 4° C – 3 h ($n = 7$); (—○—) HbPP perfusion – 3 h ($n = 7$); (--■--) sham procedure ($n = 6$)

4.1.3.1 Determination of pO_2, pCO_2, Bicarbonate, and Base Excess

In addition, random measurements of arterial pO_2, pCO_2, standard bicarbonate, and base excess were collected during reperfusion as data for future studies and hypothesis formation. The mean values with standard deviation are presented in Fig. 11.

4.1.3.2 Washout Effect: Blood Gas Analysis

During perfusion of the neurovascular pedicle-graft canine hind limbs, samples of free-flowing efflux that had just previously passed through the ischemic vasculature were collected and subjected to blood gas analysis. The mean values and standard deviations of ten perfusion procedures are depicted in Fig. 12.

4.1.3.3 Inorganic Phosphate Levels in Serum

Inorganic phosphate levels in serum served as yet another randomly studied parameter. Within all three experiment groups during the first 6 h of the procedure, no differentiation in mean values was noted. During the reperfusion phase, however, there was a divergence of the serum levels. As a result of amputation, there was evidence of a slight increase of 7.26 ± 1.27 mg/ml in Pi concentration in all three groups. Following release of the clamps, the curve tendency shown in Fig. 13 developed.

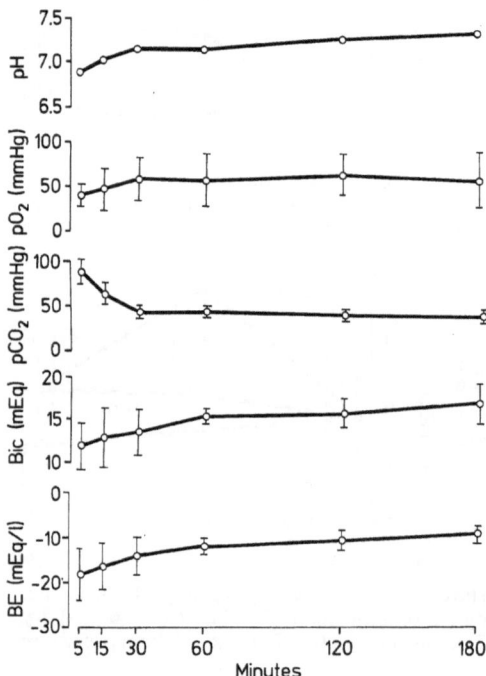

Fig. 12. Blood gas analysis of washout effect in venous efflux of canine hind limbs following 3 h of ischemia at 22° C and subsequent 3-h HbPP perfusion ($n=7$). *Bic*, bicarbonate; *BE*, base excess

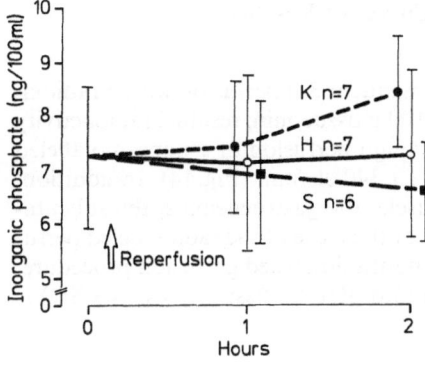

Fig. 13. Washout effect in circulating aortic blood following 3 h of ischemia at 22° C and: (---■---) dry cooling – *3 h* (*n*=7); (—○—) HbPP perfusion – *3 h* (*n*=7); (--□--) sham procedure (*n*=6)

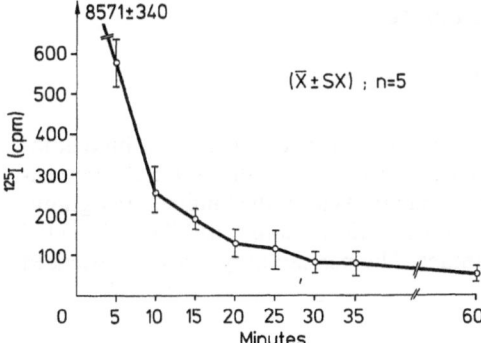

Fig. 14. Washout effect after 3 h of ischemia at 22° C followed by 3-h perfusion with a radiolabeled oxygenated HbPP solution and 1-h *non*radiolabeled HbPP perfusion (flow rate – 4 ml/100 g tissue weight/min, counts ^{125}I-labeled HbPP in venous efflux)

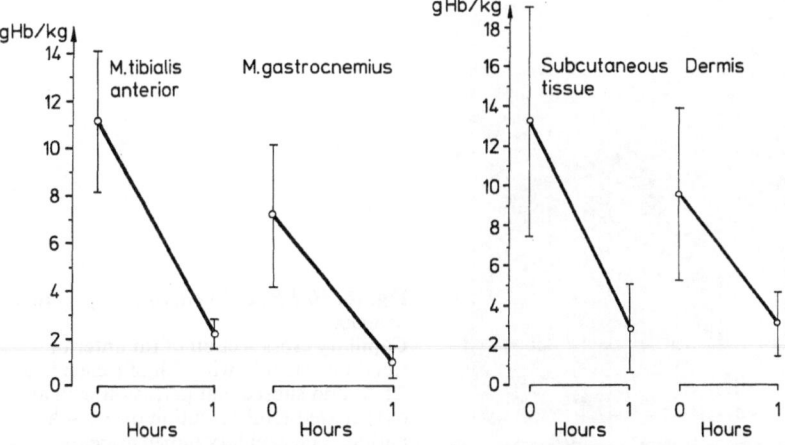

Fig. 15. Residual quantitative analysis of various tissues within the canine hind limb. Following 3 h of ischemia at 22° C, 3-h perfusion with a radiolabeled HbPP solution was performed with subsequent 1-h perfusion employing a *non*radiolabeled HbPP solution (given as g Hb/kg tissue weight, converted from the counts of ^{125}I-labeled HbPP per weight units; *n*=5; X±SX)

4.1.3.4 Washout Effect and Descending Curves of Residua with ^{125}I-labeled HbPP Solution

Following 3 h of ischemia at 22° C and subsequent 3-h perfusion with a radiolabeled HbPP solution at a flow rate of 4 ml/100 g tissue/min, residual radioactivity was measured within the venous efflux through perfusion of a nonradiolabeled HbPP solution. The exit baseline was 8571 ± 340 cts/min (Fig. 14). In addition, tissue samples from the anterior tibial muscle, the gastrocnemius, the subcutaneous tissue, and the dermis were collected at the close of the radiolabeled perfusion procedure as well as at the end of the nonradiolabeled perfusion procedure. The conversion of the radioactive cts/min into gHb/kg tissue ($n = 4$, $X \pm SD$) is shown in Fig. 15.

4.2 Histomorphology and Ultrastructure

4.2.1 Electron-Optical Results in Rat Hind-Limb Musculature

Following 2 h of ischemia at 22° C and subsequent 4-h perfusion of the hind limbs with an oxygenated HbPP solution, the capillaries of the anterior tibial compartment demonstrated good flow-through capacity. Within the lumina, gray granulated material was found (possibly fixated hemoglobin solution). The endothelial cells and basal membranes remained intact. The pericapillary space experienced a slight edema (Fig. 16).

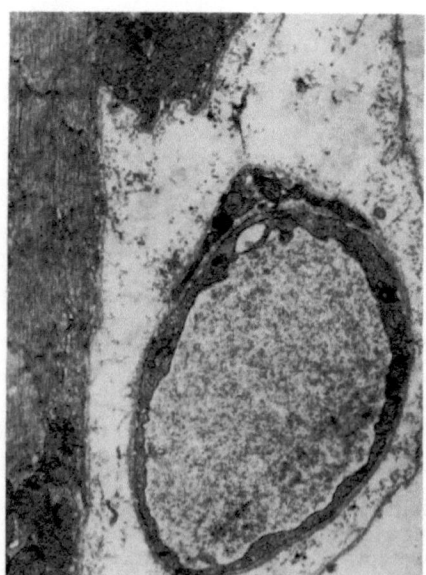

Fig. 16. *HbPP perfusion, rat, 4 h perfusion, ×8000.*
Capillary cross section of rat anterior tibial muscle following 2 h of ischemia at 22° C and subsequent perfusion with an oxygenated HbPP solution over a 4-h period. The capillary lumen appears unobstructed, and gray granulated material can be seen (possibly fixated HbPP solution). Endothelial cells and basal membrane remain intact. Only a slight pericapillary edema is observable

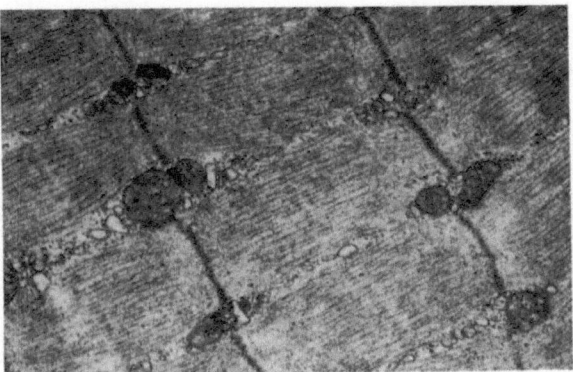

Fig. 17. *HbPP perfusion, rat, 4 h perfusion, × 12000.*
Skeletal muscle fiber specimen from rat anterior tibial muscle. Experimental procedure same as that described in Figure 16. Along with regular myofibrillar structure, a normal endoplasmic reticulum, and granules of glycogen, an intact intramitochondrial cristae architecture can be seen

Muscle samples from the anterior tibial compartment of the rat showed regular muscle fiber structure. Along with a normal endoplasmic reticulum and an intact intramitochondrial cristae structure, glycogen granules were observed (Fig. 17).

4.2.2 Photomicroscopical Studies in Canine Models

4.2.2.1 Dry-Cooling Group

A 3-h ischemic period at 22° C followed by 3-h hypothermic storage at 4° C led to a reproducible severe reperfusion injury within the muscle cells. Subtotal necrosis of the muscle fibers was pronounced 24–48 h following declamping. The striation of the muscle cells had totally diminished and numerous fibers showed a fractured sarcoplasm. The endomysial interstitial space appeared distended and severely edematous (Fig. 18).

Overall, the lesions within the anterior tibial muscle were far more severe than those involving the medial head of the gastrocnemius muscle. As many as 70% of the anterior tibial muscle fibers were destroyed, while only 20%–30% of the muscle fibers within the gastrocnemius were. Up until the 5th–6th postoperative day, group-specific alterations were seen. Necrotic and fractured skeletal muscle fibers were still observed, but no calcification or infiltration of granulocytes could be found. Within the endomysium during this period, an increasingly dense infiltration of macrophages and fibroblasts could be traced. The macrophages entered the fiber through the sarcolemmal sheaths and phagocytosed the necrotic degradation products. In many cases the sarcolemma remained intact (Fig. 19).

Within the interstitial space the fibroblasts located themselves parallel to the remaining sarcoplasmic tubes. Between the fibroblasts were myoblasts with eccentrically positioned nuclei possessing pronounced nucleoli (Fig. 20).

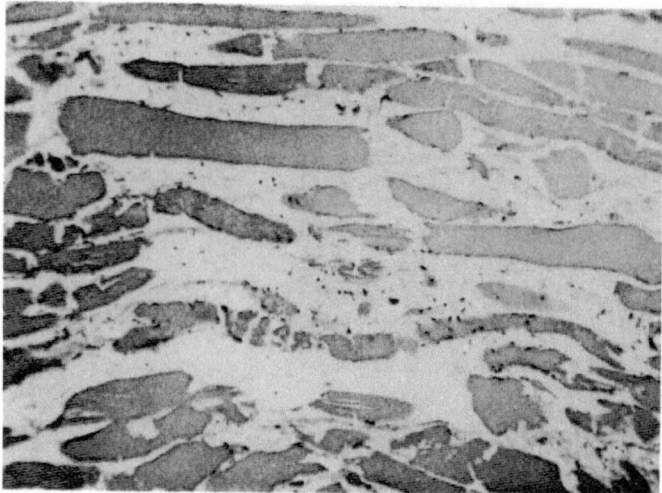

Fig. 18. *Dry cooling, canine, 24 h after operation, H and E, × 250.*
Muscle sample taken from canine anterior tibial site following 3 h of storage at 22° C and
subsequent 3 h hypothermic storage at 4° C; 24–48 h following declamping, necrotic
muscle cells with pyknotic nuclei are markedly pronounced. The striation of the muscle
cells is gone and numerous fibers show a fractured sarcoplasmic structure. Severe edema
and enduring sarcolemmal sheaths are observable

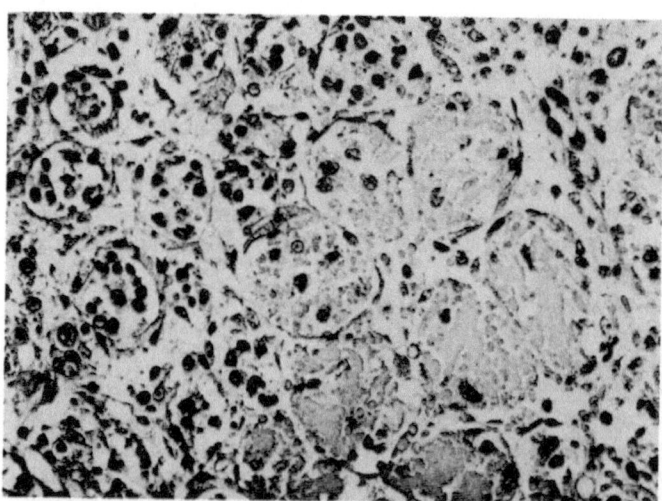

Fig. 19. *Dry cooling, canine, 5 days after operation, H and E, × 400.*
Anterior tibial muscle sample harvested following the same experimental procedure as that
described in Fig. 18. On the 5th postoperative day necrosis and fracturing of the muscle
fibers is still observable. An increase in dense infiltration of macrophagocytes and fibroblasts can be seen. The macrophages enter the fiber through the sarcolemmal sheath and
phagocytose the necrotic degradation products

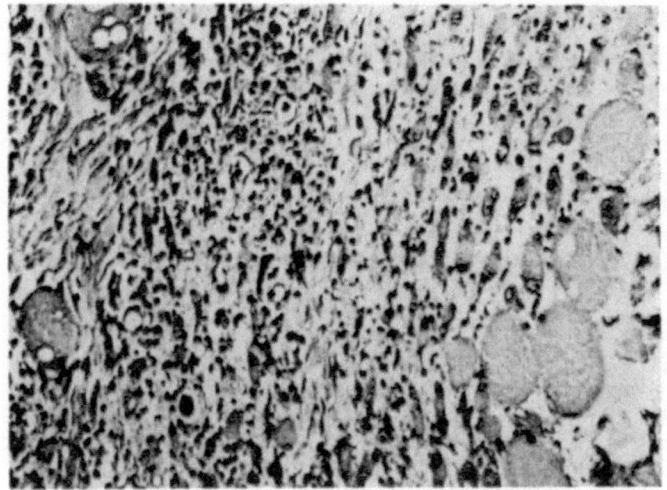

Fig. 20. *Dry cooling, canine, 6 days after operation, H and E, × 250.*
Tissue sample from canine anterior tibial muscle following the same experimental procedure as that described in Fig. 18. On the 6th postoperative day fibroblasts have located themselves parallel to the remaining sarcoplasmic tubes. Between the fibroblasts are myoblasts with eccentrically positioned nuclei possessing pronounced nucleoli

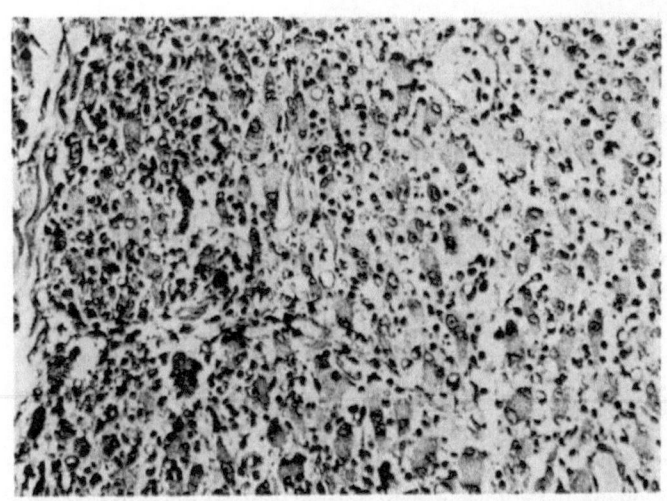

Fig. 21. *Dry cooling, canine, 8 days after operation, H and E, × 250.*
Tissue sample taken from canine anterior tibial muscle on the 8th postoperative day; myoblastic structures exhibit a higher intensity. A few regenerated muscle fibers are observable with enlarged nuclei (myotubes) and markedly reduced calibers

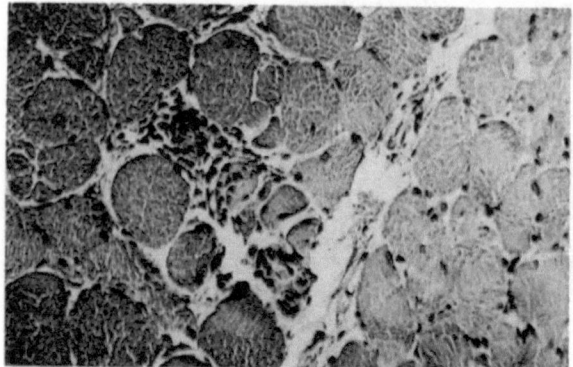

Fig. 22. *Dry cooling, canine, 3 months after operation, H and E, ×400.*
Canine anterior tibial muscle. Three months following the same procedure as with sample in Fig. 21, almost normal skeletal musculature can be seen. The young fibers, however are clearly narrower and have slightly enlarged nuclei. Within the endomysial stroma there are aggregations of macrophages and fibroblasts

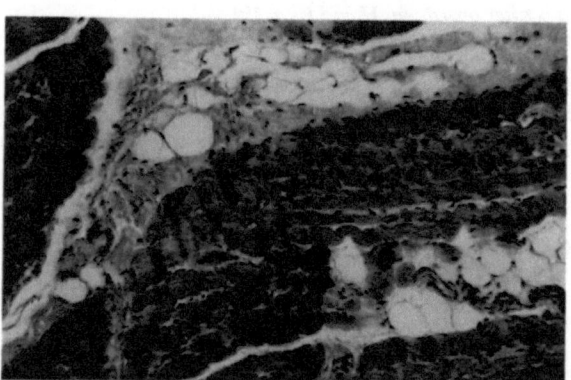

Fig. 23. *Dry cooling, canine, 3 months after operation, H and E, ×250.*
Canine anterior tibial muscle, 3 months post-op. Within the perimysium small and large areas of scarring containing collagenous connective tissue can be seen. Scattered congregations of metaplastic macrovacuolar fatty tissue are also noted. Variations in muscle fiber caliber remain

On the 8th postoperative day the myoblastic structures were more intense. Regenerated muscle fibers with enlarged nuclei (myotubes) and markedly reduced in caliber were sparse. Once again, the lesions within the anterior tibial musculature were seen to be far more severe than those within the gastrocnemius muscle (Fig. 21).

Three months following the studies nearly normal skeletal musculature was observed with parallel muscle fibers. These young fibers were clearly narrower than normal muscle cell fibers and frequently had a sharply angular shape with enlarged nuclei. Within the endomysial stroma were intermittently defined areas of macrophages and fibroblasts (Fig. 22).

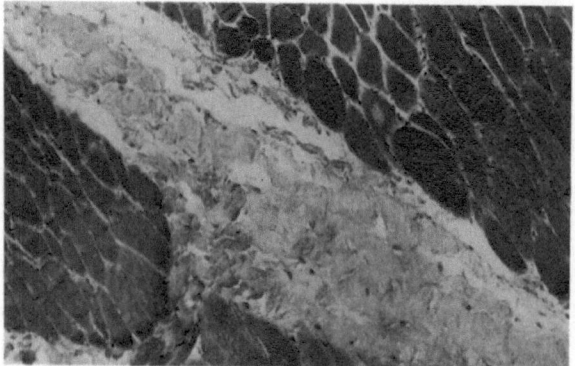

Fig. 24. *Dry cooling, canine, 1.5 years after operation, H and E, × 100.*
Sample taken from canine anterior tibial muscle 1.5 years after 3 h of storage at 22° C and subsequent 3 h of hypothermic storage at 4° C. The muscle consists mainly of regularly organized fiber bundles, but there are persistent areas of scarring. Along with variations in caliber, the fibers often exhibit angulated borders

Within this time period small and large areas of scar tissue with collagenous connective tissue were seen within the perimysium. In addition, scattered congregations of metaplastic fatty tissue were noted. Within the cross sections there existed a marked variation in muscle fiber caliber (Fig. 23).

From 3 months to 1.5 years postoperatively, no further changes could be observed photomicroscopically. The regenerated muscle showed a normal parallel structure. Certain muscle bundles, however, remained characterized by small or large areas of scar tissue or by deposits of fat cells.

Along with persistent variations in caliber, the muscle fibers frequently exhibited angulated borders. Remaining injuries to the anterior tibial muscle were, as before, more severe than those to the gastrocnemius muscle of the same limb (Fig. 24).

4.2.2.2 HbPP Perfusion Group

Following a 3-h ischemic period at 22° C and subsequent 3-h perfusion with an oxygenated HbPP solution, this experimental group exhibited principally the same injuries as those occurring in the other groups; however, these injuries were quantitatively far less pronounced.

Scattered aggregations of single cell necrosis appeared exclusively within the anterior tibial muscle 24 and 48 h following reperfusion of the limb with systemic circulation. Although approximately 10% of the fibers within the anterior tibial muscle were found to be necrotic, necrosis was totally absent within the gastrocnemius muscle. As was the case with the dry-cooling group, decomposition of the skeletal musculature did take place – however, without calcification or accompanying granulocytic infiltration (Fig. 25). Within the region of necrosis a moderate interstitial edema developed.

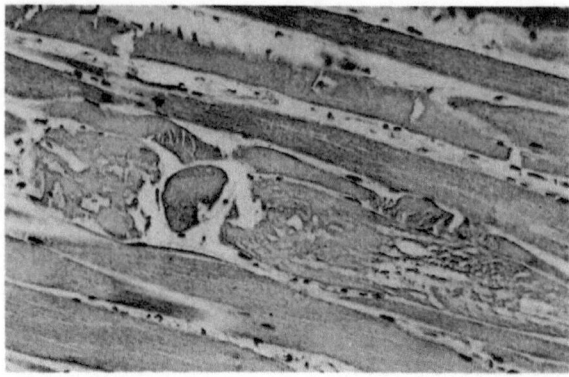

Fig. 25. *HbPP perfusion, canine, 48 h after operation, H and E, ×400.*
Muscle sample taken from canine anterior tibial site 48 h following 3 h of ischemia at 22° C
and subsequent 3-h perfusion with an oxygenated HbPP solution. In contrast to the dry-
cooling group, only a moderate interstitial edema is noted, along with minor aggregations
of single cell necrosis

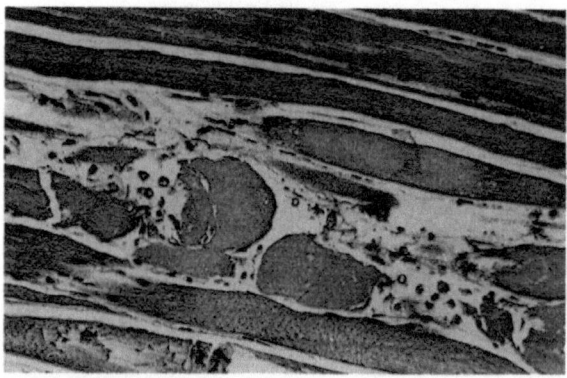

Fig. 26. *HbPP perfusion, canine, 6 days after operation, H and E, ×400.*
Muscle sample taken from canine anterior tibial site 6 days post-op, following the same
procedures as described in Fig. 25. A decrease in interstitial edema is evident, as macrophages phagocytose degradation products found within the sarcolemmal sheath

Up to the 5th–8th postoperative day, reparative processes were evident within
isolated areas of muscle cell necrosis. This was quite similar to the course undergone by the dry cooling group, in that the macrophages phagocytosed the necrotic degradation products (Fig. 26).

Within the interstitial space appeared very few proliferating fibroblasts and
myoblasts. Quite similar to the initial necrotic aggregations, these injuries were
clearly more pronounced within the anterior tibial muscle but absent within the
region of the gastrocnemius muscle (Fig. 27). Three months to 1.5 years postoperatively, the regenerated muscle displayed no histomorphological changes.

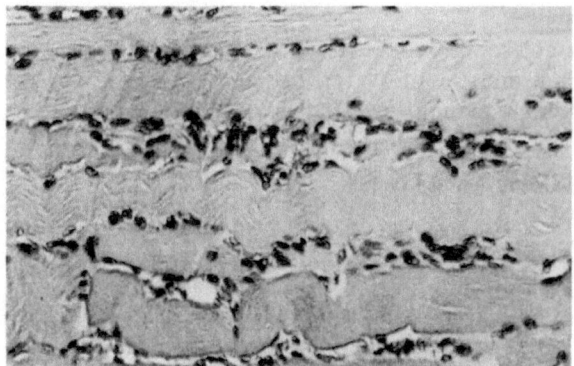

Fig. 27. *HbPP perfusion, canine, 8 days after operation, H and E, × 250.*
Muscle sample taken from canine anterior tibial site 8 days following the same procedure described in Fig. 25. Within the interstitial space, very few proliferating fibroblasts and myoblasts are observed

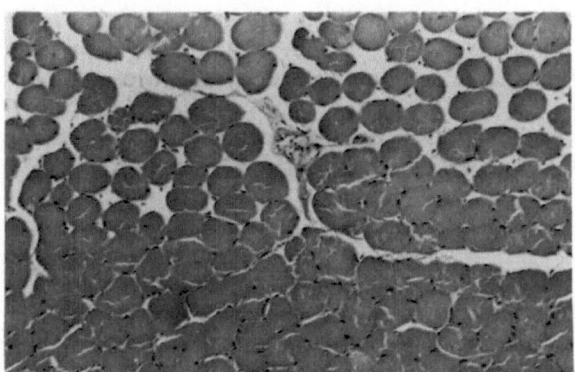

Fig. 28. *HbPP perfusion, canine, 1.5 years after operation, H and E, × 100.*
Muscle sample taken from canine anterior tibial site 1.5 years following the same procedure as described in Fig. 25. In contrast to those in the dry-cooling group, fibers show no variations in caliber or diameter, nor do they exhibit areas of scar tissue or fatty metaplasia

Muscle fiber diameters proved to be normal and no variations in caliber were seen. In contrast to the dry-cooling group however, no areas of scar tissue or metaplastic fatty tissue were seen (Fig. 28).

4.2.2.3 Sham Procedure Group

After preparation of the hind-limb neurovascular pedicle, intimal lesions to the femoral vein and artery were produced by means of short-term clamping and vascular angiorrhaphy. Following a procedure otherwise identical to that for the other groups, no histomorphological changes developed within the musculature.

4.2.2.4 Contralateral Extremities

Within all three groups samples were collected not only from the anterior tibial muscle and gastrocnemius muscles of the rejoined limbs but also from the contralateral unoperated limb. No pathological changes or injuries were noted.

4.2.3 Histological Studies of Kidneys and Livers

4.2.3.1 Dry-Cooling Group

Within a 24- to 48-h time period following 3 h of ischemia at 22° C and subsequent storage at 4° C, kidneys and livers of the dry-cooling group showed diserect signs of compensated shock syndrome. The renal tubules were slightly distended and often contained sparse tracings of myoglobin.

Sporadic incidences of isolated centrilobular single-cell necrosis were seen within the livers, but no further injuries to the organs were observed.

4.2.3.2 HbPP Perfusion Group

In contrast to those of the dry-cooling group, livers and kidneys of the HbPP perfusion group showed normal structure. Renal tubules were minimally distended and no signs of hemoglobin excretion were detectable with photomicroscopy.

The livers showed only congested sinuses within the lobular centers, and in the ensuing months (up to 1.5 years) no traces of hemosiderin were found.

4.2.3.3 Sham Procedure Group

The liver and kidney specimens from this group showed no pathological signs of change at any point postoperatively.

4.2.4 Electron-Optical Studies in Dogs

4.2.4.1 Dry-Cooling Group

On the 1st and 2nd days following 3 h of ischemia at 22° C and subsequent hypothermic storage of the hind limbs, all phenomena related to severe ischemic muscle cell damage became clearly apparent (Fig. 29). Along with intense edematous swelling and vacuolar degeneration of the sarcoplasmic reticulum, the muscle fibers exhibited disruption of the myofibrillar structures with still-existing transverse striation. Condensation of the myofibrils resulted with a decline in transverse striation and an increase in osmophilia (Fig. 30). Eventually, cells with irregular fine-fiber coagulation necrosis of the sarcoplasma appeared, accompanied by severely swollen mitochondria and overwhelming destruction of the crystae architecture, vacuolation, and trilaminated structures.

During this phase, the majority of the capillaries demonstrated cystically swollen endothelium with more than 50% obstruction of the lumina. In addition, the pericapillary space exhibited marked edema (Fig. 31).

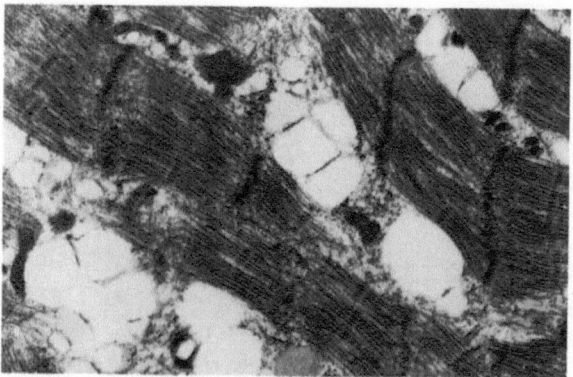

Fig. 29. *Dry cooling, canine, 24 h after operation, × 10000.*
Severe ischemic muscle cell damage in the dog 24 h following 3-h normothermic storage
at 22° C and subsequent 3-h hypothermic storage at 4° C. Intense edematous swelling with
vacuolated degeneration of the sarcoplasmic reticulum is seen, along with disruption of the
basic myofibrillar structure. Transverse striation of the fibers is still evident at this point

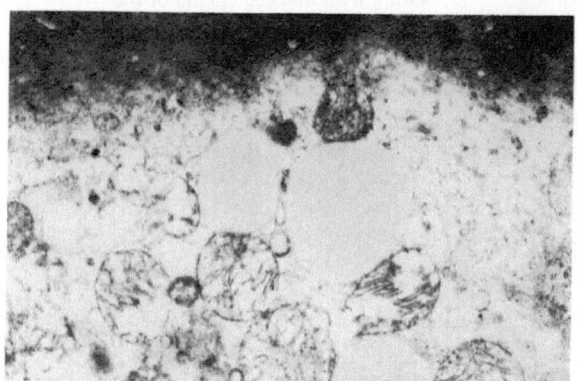

Fig. 30. *Dry cooling, canine, 24 h after operation, × 8000.*
Twenty-four hours following the procedure described in Fig. 29, zones of condensed myofibrils are evident resulting in a disappearance of transverse striation and an increase in osmophilia. Irregular fine-filament coagulation necrosis of the sarcoplasma accompanied by
severely swollen mitochondria and overwhelming destruction of the cristae architecture,
along with vacuolation and trilaminated structures

Within the areas of high-grade swelling and partially destroyed endothelium
developed multifocal clots of erythrocyte and thrombocyte adhesion (Fig. 32).
Pericapillary edema was also present, with fragmentation of the sarcoplasmic reticulum.

In parallel to the histomorphological findings, large areas of muscle fiber necrosis were noted up to the 6th postoperative day. Also, within the photomicroscopically examined intact areas, ultrastructural pathological injuries were found.
Numerous muscle fibers showed localized areas of partial or complete fibrilloly-

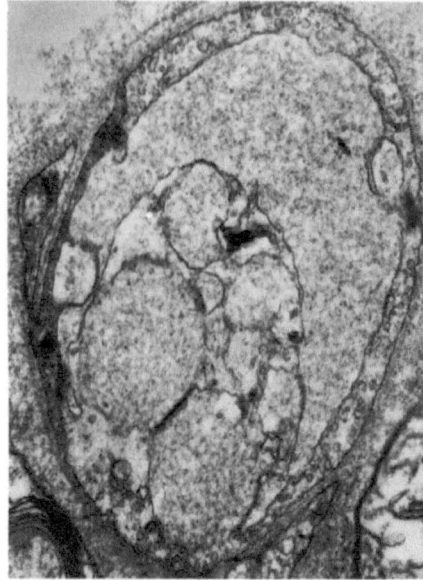

Fig. 31. *Dry cooling, canine, 24 h after operation, × 9000.*
Capillary cross section from canine anterior tibial muscle 24 h following 3 h of storage at 22° C and subsequent 3-h hypothermic storage at 4° C. A cystically swollen endothelium with more than 50% obstruction of the lumina can be seen, along with marked edema of the pericapillary space

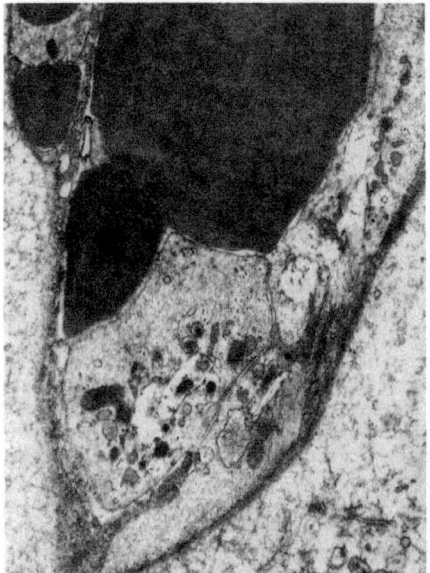

Fig. 32. *Dry cooling, canine, 24 h after operation, × 12000.*
Capillary cross section 24 h following the same procedure as described in Fig. 31. Areas of high-grade swelling, partial destruction of the endothelial lining, and clot formations of erythrocyte and thrombocyte adhesions have developed. Marked pericapillary edema is observable, along with fragments of the sarcoplasmic reticulum

sis. Partial fibrillolysis was accompanied by diminution of thin actin filaments and persistence of the thicker myosin filaments (Fig. 33).

At this stage, the intramitochondrial regeneration processes had almost completely reestablished the cristae architecture. Within the zones of complete fibrillolysis a complete absence of muscle fibril remnants was noted. Around the mar-

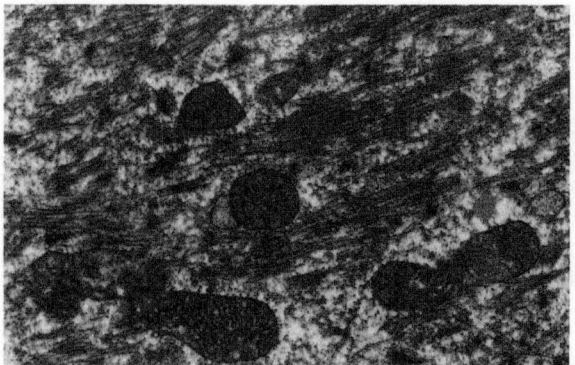

Fig. 33. *Dry cooling, canine, 5 days after operation,* × *10 000.*
Sample from canine anterior tibial muscle 5 days following 3 h of storage at 22° C and subsequent 3-h hypothermic storage at 4° C. Ultrastructural pathological injuries are observable. Localized areas of partial or complete fibrillolysis result in a dimunition of thin actin
filaments and persistence of thicker myosin filaments. At this point in time, already regenerating intramitochondrial basic structural elements can be seen

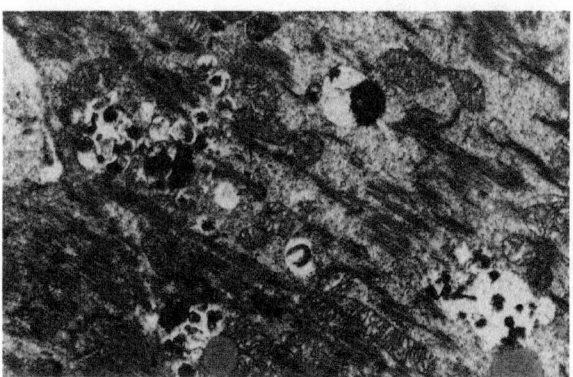

Fig. 34. *Dry cooling, canine, 5 days after operation,* × *6000.*
Muscle tissue sample from canine anterior tibial site 5 days following the same procedure
as described in Fig. 33. Within the areas of complete fibrillolysis, muscle fibrils are absent.
Within the borders large intracellular phagolysosomes are seen

ginal areas appeared large intracellular phagolysosomes (Fig. 34). These same
phagolysosomes were detectable months later as lipofuscin particles within the
marginal areas of the fibers.

Three months after the conclusion of the experiments, the muscles studied
continued to demonstrate single fibers with persistently localized areas of focal
fibrillolysis. In this area, along with otherwise normal cell organelles, severely distorted mitochondria appeared quite often. Z-band material in an atypical arrangement with intact sarcoplasmic reticulum was present as well (Fig. 35).

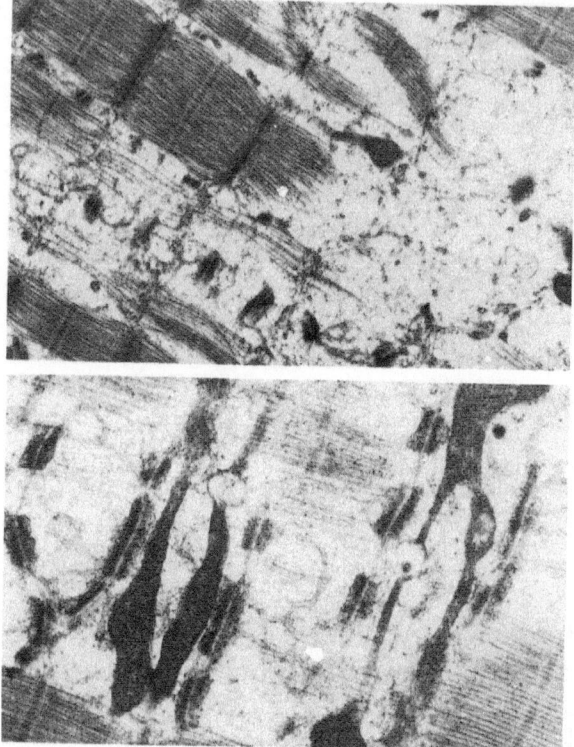

Fig. 35 a, b. *Dry cooling, canine, 3 months after operation.* **a** × 9000; **b** × 14000.
Muscle tissue samples taken from canine anterior tibial site 3 months following the procedure described in Fig. 33. Isolated fibers with localized areas of focal fibrillolysis persist. Along with apparently normal cell organelles, severely distorted mitochondria are often found. Z-band material in an atypical arrangement with intact sarcoplasmic reticulum is also present

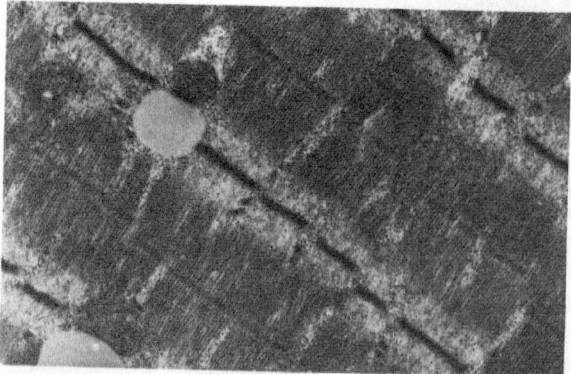

Fig. 36. *Dry cooling, canine, 1.5 years after operation,* × 10000.
Muscle tissue sample from canine anterior tibial site 1.5 years following the procedure described in Fig. 33. Regularly formed muscle fibers containing lipid deposits and regenerated mitochondria are seen

One and a half years following ischemic injury to the hind limbs, electron-optical studies uncovered regularly formed muscle fibers containing lipid deposits as evidence of previous lesions (Fig. 36).

4.2.4.2 HbPP Perfusion Group

In contrast to the dry-cooling group, the HbPP perfusion group (3 h of ischemia at 22° C and subsequent 3-h HbPP perfusion) postoperatively exhibited only localized necrotic muscle fibers 24–48 h. Figure 37 clearly shows an area within the anterior tibial compartment of partially dispersed and partially condensed internal structure. Small intramuscular capillaries showed structurally normal cell wall

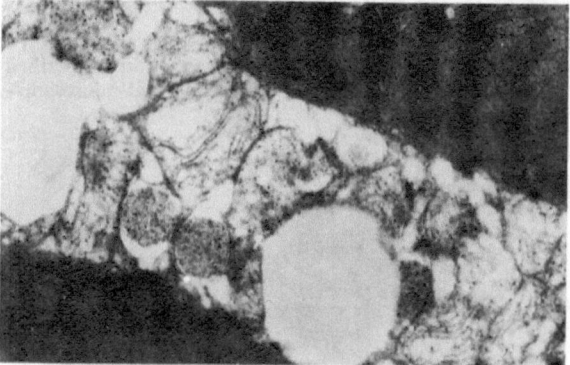

Fig. 37. *HbPP perfusion, canine, 48 h after operation,* × *14 000.*
Forty-eight hours following 3 h storage at 22° C and subsequent 3-h perfusion with an oxygenated HbPP solution, tissue sample taken from canine anterior tibial muscle demonstrates only localized necrotic muscle fibers with partially dispersed and partially condensed internal structure

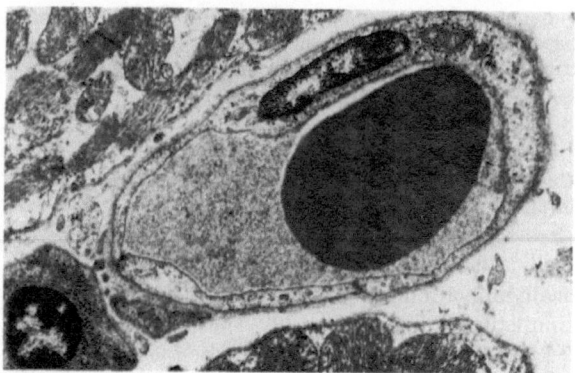

Fig. 38. *HbPP perfusion, canine, 48 h after operation,* × *6000.*
Capillary cross section from canine anterior tibial site 48 h following procedure described in Fig. 37. Note structurally normal cell wall and unobstructed lumina. There is also slight pericapillary and intracellular edema with isolated incidences of myofibrillar disruption but generally intact mitochondrial structures

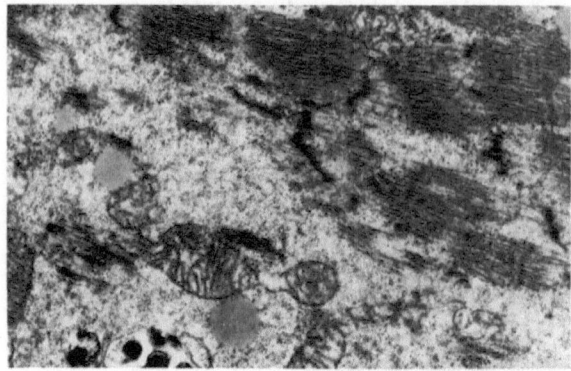

Fig. 39. *HbPP perfusion, canine, 8 days after operation,* × *10 000.*
Muscle tissue sample from canine anterior tibial site 8 days following procedure described in Fig. 37. Zones of partial or complete fibrillolysis are seen in areas of light-microscopically intact muscle fibers

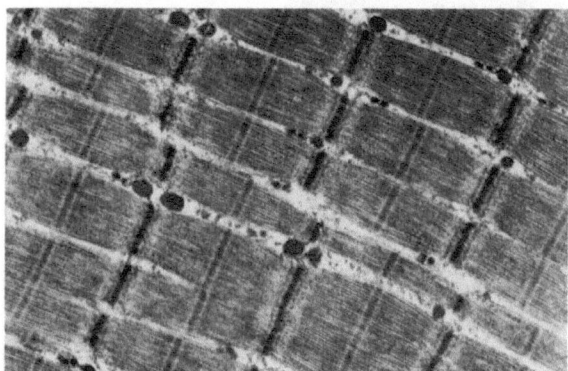

Fig. 40. *HbPP perfusion, canine, 3 months after operation,* × *9000.*
Muscle tissue sample taken from the canine anterior tibial site 3 months following procedures identical to those described in Fig. 37. In contrast to the dry-cooling group, no essential ultrastructural changes are evident on this longitudinal section

formation as well as unobstructed lumina. Also noted within the area were mitochondria with regular cristae structure.

There was as well evidence of slight pericapillary and intracellular edema with isolated incidences of myofibrillar disruption (Fig. 38). During the first postoperative week, photomicroscopically intact muscle fibers were also found to display partial and in some places complete fibrillolysis (Fig. 39). These fibers contained isolated fat deposits as well as phagolysosomes with intact mitochondrial internal structure.

After 3 months, in contrast to the dry-cooling group, the hind limbs within the HbPP perfusion group exhibited no essential ultrastructural muscle fiber in-

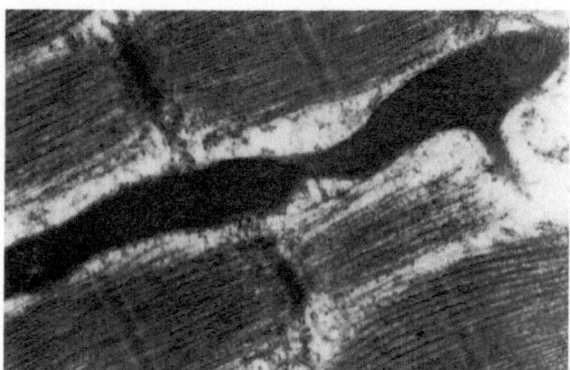

Fig. 41. *HbPP perfusion, canine, 3 months after operation, × 15 000.*
Muscle tissue sample taken from the canine anterior tibial site 3 months following the procedure described in Fig. 37. Under higher magnification, such unusually shaped mitochondrial structures are rarely seen

juries (Fig. 40). The persistent areas of fibrillolysis found in the hind-limb musculature of the dry-cooling group were *not* observed in the HbPP perfusion group. However, unusually formed tubular mitochondria were evident within some specimens (Fig. 41).

4.2.4.3 Sham Procedure Group

The skeletal musculature of the hind limbs following establishment of a neurovascular pedicle hind-limb graft, including intimal injury to the femoral vein and artery, yielded no abnormal electron-optical findings.

5 Discussion

5.1 Major and Minor Limb Replantation

Although reports of the first successful replantations of completely severed arms date back as far as 1962 (Malt 1964 and 1963; Chen et al. 1981), major limb replantation has not achieved routine procedure status, owing mainly to the occurrence of complications such as renal failure, pulmonary insufficiency (ARDS), septicemia, clotting disorders, and even death as a direct result of postischemia syndrome (Ferreira et al. 1978; Matsuda et al. 1978; May and Gallico 1980; Baudet 1981; Coonrad and Milford 1981; Chen et al. 1981; Berger 1983; Doi et al. 1983; Piza et al. 1983; Russel 1985; Maurer et al. 1986).

In sharp contrast, minor replantations such as of fingers and hand portions have increased markedly, despite relatively late introduction of meticulous microsurgical techniques. The experimental procedures carried out and reported by Jacobson (1962) and Kleinert and Kasdan (1963) helped lead to the first successful replantation of an amputated thumb by Komatsu and Tamai in 1965 (1968). In the meantime, minor limb replantation has become a routine undertaking at specialized plastic surgery centers, yielding take rates of more than 80% (O'Brien and McLeod 1976; Biemer 1977; Biemer and Duspiva 1982; Tamai et al. 1979; Tamai 1984; Kleinert et al. 1980; May and Gallico 1980; Chen 1981; Wang et al. 1981; Tamai 1982). Even in the case of detachment, segmental crush, or degloving injury, successful reconstruction can be accomplished through the use of microvenous interpositional grafts (O'Brien 1977; Biemer 1977; Biemer and Duspiva 1982; Yoshizu et al. 1978; Kleinert et al. 1980; Chen et al. 1981).

The reattachment of extremities possessing predominantly muscular tissue, however, all too frequently presents life-threatening complications, the analysis of which is difficult, because of several factors:

1. Statistical review and interpretation of the available data is severely hindered and quite often impossible because differing amputation levels are reported and misleading information is published by various authors on patients from the same collective (Williams 1966; McNeill and Wilson 1970; Engber 1971; Sixth People's Hospital Shanghai 1975; Coonrad and Milford 1981; Chen 1981; Koch et al. 1981; Zwank 1981; Zwank and Eckert 1983).
2. Evaluation of satisfactory end results is made difficult by variations in periods of warm or cold ischemia, the degree of crush injury, age differences, additional injury to the remainder of the body as a whole, the art and frequency of secondary procedures found to be necessary during the rehabilitation period, the quality of physical therapy provided, and, last but not least, the compliance of the patient.

3. Attempts at major limb replantation unfortunately often go unreported when they lead to forced primary or secondary reamputation, unsatisfactory end results, or death.

It must also be mentioned, however, that despite the number of frustrating failures that have occurred, there is an impressive list of accomplishments. A review of the data on 274 arm replantations (at several differing levels) revealed a success rate of 80%–95% with patients suffering from hand or distal forearm amputation (Morrison et al. 1977; Ikuta 1978; Matsuda et al. 1978; Manke et al. 1980; Nunley et al. 1981; Coonrad and Milford 1981; Wang et al. 1981; Tamai 1982; Chen et al. 1982), while procedures performed in the upper arm region had 50%–80% positive results (Chung Shan 1973; Chishueit'an 1975; Ikuta 1978; Maurer et al. 1979; Coonrad and Milford 1981; Chen et al. 1982).

For the 54 cases of leg replantation cited within the literature, an average success rate of only 50% can be claimed, due mainly to severe concomitant crush injuries (Chung Shan 1973; Chishueit'an 1975; Sixth People's Hospital Shanghai 1975; Zwank et al. 1980a; Zwank and Eckert 1983; Coonrad and Milford 1981; Berger 1983; Chen et al. 1982; Maurer et al. 1986).

Without question, only those cases of limb replantation that clearly provide some degree of functional restoration can be interpreted as truly successful. According to the guidelines of Carroll's Extremity Function Evaluation Scores (1965), a *useful limb* must be the goal of every replantation attempt (Chase 1970; Malt et al. 1972; Buri 1973; O'Brien and McLeod 1976; Kleinert et al. 1980; Zwank et al. 1980; Rüter and Burri 1981; Beasley 1981; Brown 1981). Similar functional criteria have been postulated by Horn (1969), Malt et al. (1972), Morrison et al. (1977), Coonrad and Milford (1981), Chen et al. (1982), and Maurer et al. (1986), with reintegration at a place of work and routine daily use of the replanted limb as parameters of success.

In interesting contrast to the course of events in minor limb replantation, major limb replantation remains a risky undertaking, despite advances in technical procedures such as angiorrhaphy, tenorraphy, neurorraphy, muscle suture, external/internal bone fixation, physiotherapy, orthotic devices, and intensive perioperative care. The potential for failure has therefore been assumed to be closely dependent upon the degree of ischemia-induced injury within limb tissues.

5.2 Perfusion, Storage, and Pharmacological Treatment of Postischemia Syndrome

To date, numerous variations on pharmacological therapies as well as perfusion and storage methods have been recommended and tried as means of avoiding local ischemic lesion or postischemia syndrome (see Table 5). Experiments on various species, with various tissue types, and under varying ischemic periods produced differing and often contradictory data. Perfusion using a heart-lung machine and employing oxygenated full blood was performed in an effort to simulate autogenous circulation (Lapchinski 1960; Letac et al. 1963; Synder 1963; Onji et al. 1963; Delorme et al. 1964; Stipa et al. 1967; Kowanow et al. 1968). For clinical

Table 5. Storage and perfusion methods for preventing postischemia syndrome

Author	Year	Method	Duration (h)	Species and tissue type
Allen	1938	Cooling, 2° C	55.5	Rat, dog, cat hind limb
Lapchinski	1954– 1960	Full blood oxygenator, hypothermia at 2°–4° C	28	Dog, hind limb
Letac et al.	1963	Oxygenated blood	4–6	Dog, hind limb
Snyder	1963	Full blood oxygenator	8	Dog, hind limb
Onji et al.	1963	Full blood oxygenator	6	Dog, hind limb
Eiken et al.	1964	Dextran solution, isotonic salt solution	3.5	Dog, hind limb
Mehl et al.	1964a, b	0.9% NaCl with and without heparin, 5% dextrose and rheomacrodex, 5% dextrose with thrombolysin, buffer solution, hyper-thermia at 10° C and 2° C	21.5	Dog, hind limb
Hamel and Moe	1964	Hypothermia at 18° C, 13° C, 10° C, −2° C	5	Dog, hind limb
Delorme et al.	1964	Full blood recalcified, dextran	5	Man, amputated extremities
Stipa et al.	1967	Full blood, THAM, Rheo	10	Dog, hind limb
Kowanow et al.	1968	Oxygenator, 18°–20° C	24	Dog, hind limb
Strock et al.	1968	Homologous plasma, Ringer's lactate-heparin	5.5	Dog, hind limb
Sixth People's Hospital Shanghai	1967, 1975	NaCl with heparin, hypothermia at 4° C, HBO	108	Dog, fore limb and hind limb
Brückner	1972	Allopurinol hypoxanthine	5	Dog, hind limb
Strohfeld	1973	Bovine albumin, erythrocytes pyruvate, glucose, Krebs-Henseleit solution	3	Rat, hind limb (low-flow)
O'Connell et al.	1974	Physiological saline	1–3	Rabbit carotid artery
Stock et al.	1974	Mg-aspartase	5	Dog, hind limb
Hayhurst et al.	1974	Hypothermia at 4° C	24	Large primate, fingers
Harashina and Buncke	1975	Isotonic salt solution with heparin, Collin's solution, hypothermia at 4° C	5.5	Rat, hind limb

Table 5. (Continued)

Author	Year	Method	Duration (h)	Species and tissue type
Stock et al.	1976	Collin's solution, hypothermia at 4° C	10	Dog, hind limb
Monies-Chass et al.	1977	HBO	20	Man, lower extremities
Usui et al.	1978	Dry and wet cooling	12	Dog, hind limb
Chait et al.	1978	Hartmann solution with heparin mannitol, cortisone	12	Rabbit, epigastric flaps
Steinau et al.	1979	Stroma-free hemoglobin	6–8	Rat, dog, man, amputated extremities
Smahel	1979	Solcoseryl	15	Rat, hind limb
Hicks et al.	1980	Collin's solution dextran-dextrose, Ringer's lactate, and hypothermia at 4° C	20	Rat, hind limb
Eisenhard et al.	1980	Hypothermia at 4° C	4	Rat, hind limb
Tauber et al.	1981	Fluosol and hypothermia at 4° C	4	Rabbit, hind limb
Schindler	1981	Fluosol and hypothermia at 4° C	8	Rat, hind limb
Pennig and Brug	1982	Hypothermia	6	Rat, hind limb
Tsai et al.	1982	Collin's solution, hypothermia at 4° C	192	Dog, latissimus dorsi
Kaufmann and Hurwitz	1983	Hyperbaric oxygenation	42	Rat, skin flaps
Karbowski et al.	1983	Fluorocarbons	8	Rat, hind limb
Hild	1983	Stroma-free hemoglobin solution, FDA 20	1	Dog, hind limb
Usui et al.	1983	FC-43 immersion	24	Rat, epigastric flap
Imatami et al.	1984	Isotonic saline, coumarin, indomethacin, aspirin imidazole, hypothermia	72	Rabbit, groin flaps
Richt et al.	1984	FC 43	4.5	Rabbit, hind limbs
Kessler et al.	1984	Hypothermia, Collin's solution, bovine serum, normosol (low-flow)	48	Rat, hind limb
Rembs et al.	1984	Bretschneider HTP solution	4	Dog, hind limb
Lindner et al.	1985	Phosphate-buffered Ringer's solution, different agents, hypothermia at 4° C	72	Rat, groin flaps

Table 5. (Continued)

Author	Year	Method	Duration (h)	Species and tissue type
Mc Namara et al.	1985	Balanced salt solution, bicarbonate, glucose, glucogen, heparin (low-flow)		Rat, artery
Smith et al.	1985	Fluosol DA 20%, 5° C	45	Man, amputated extremities
Tsai et al.	1985	Perfluorocarbons, 20% Collin's solution, cooling	72	Dog, limbs
Rosen et al.	1985	Preischemic washout solution containing 70 trace substances	24	Rat, epigastric flaps and hind limbs
Clothiaux et al.	1985	Aerated 0.9 saline solution, 20°–24° C $\alpha 1$ and $\alpha 2$ blockers	24	Dog, tibia
Muramatsu et al.	1985	Heparin-saline washout solution, hypothermia	12	Dog, hind limb
Mailänder et al.	1985	Stroma-free hemoglobin solution		Man, finger
Mazer et al.	1986	Saline, Ringer's RTV cortisone	0.5	Rat, femoral artery
Menger et al.	1986	Hemodilution, dextran-60	4	Hamster, skin, muscle
Scharnagel	1986	Sack's solution, HBO	4.5	Rabbit, hind limb, clinical trial

purposes, however, such a procedure proved too costly and inconvenient, since not every suburban hospital possessed the necessary and complex equipment. A much simpler and less expensive approach was perfusion of dextran and electrolyte solutions at varying concentrations with different additives (Eiken 1964a, b; Mehl et al. 1964a, b; Sixth People's Hospital Shanghai 1964; Delorme et al. 1964; Strock et al. 1968; Stock et al. 1976; Harashina and Buncke 1975; Chait et al. 1978; Hicks et al. 1980; Tsai et al. 1982; Rembs et al. 1984; Mazer et al. 1986; Scharnagel 1986). Unfortunately, subsequent to this treatment, endothelial lesions, edema formation, and coagulation disturbances were actually found to be increased. Therefore, heparin (Mehl et al. 1964a, b; Strock et al. 1968; Harashina and Buncke 1975; Chait et al. 1978; Muramatsu et al. 1985), buffer solutions (Mehl et al. 1964a, b; Stipa et al. 1967; Larcan et al. 1973; McNamara et al. 1985), magnesium aspartate (Stock et al. 1974), mannitol (Chait et al. 1978; Rhodes et al. 1978; Shah et al. 1981; Hutton et al. 1982), bovine serum albumin (Kessler et al. 1984), cortisone (Hewitt et al. 1971; Ghussen and Stock 1979; Edfeld and Thomson 1980; Mazer et al. 1986), solcoseryl (Smahel 1982), imidazole, aspirin (Imatami et al. 1984), allopurinol (Brückner et al. 1972; Shandall et al. 1985; Im et al. 1985; Narayan et al. 1985), ATP-MgCl2, dipyramidole, pentoxifylline, dazoxiben (thromboxane blockers) (Lindner et al. 1985), and dextran 60 to produce hemodilution (Menger et al. 1986), were systemically or locally administered with differing effects. Systemically infused aprotinin (Trasylol) was shown to have a positive effect in inhibiting cellular damage caused by liberated proteolytic enzymes (Stock and Eigler 1969; Eigler 1974; Rahmer et al. 1977; Shandall et al. 1985). This claim was challenged, however, by Heugel in 1973 and once again by Molzberger et al. in 1978.

Contradictory information is available on the potential benefit of physically increased oxygen tissue tension during the ischemic phase and subsequent reperfusion period. While clinical reports (Sixth People's Hospital Shanghai 1971; Monies-Chass et al. 1977; Gutschi et al. 1981; Scharnagel 1986) presented evidence for lower edema rates and increased bacterial elimination potential, standardized experiments showed additional perfusion disturbances (Kaufmann and Hurwitz 1983). High periarteriolar pO_2 tensions will lead to shutdown of the terminal arterioles and capillary perfusion (Lindbom and Arfois 1984). Lowering the AV pressure gradient will decrease edema formation by inhibiting the reactive hyperemia. If postischemic malperfusion of the terminal vascular bed is already present, however, it will be intensified by reduced AV pressure gradients, with a subsequent rise in venular thrombus formation.

Immersion of epigastric flaps in highly O_2-saturated fluorocarbon solution (FC–43) during an ischemic period of up to 24 h had a definitely positive preservative effect (Usui et al. 1983). The results of this experiment were influenced, however, by variations in temperatures used. Conclusive findings pertaining to the benefit of hyperbaric oxygenation (HBO) can be drawn only when laboratory and clinical procedures for application have been standardized.

Interestingly, dry cooling of an extremity at 2°–4° C remains a unanimously supported prophylactic treatment method (Allen 1938; Lapchinski 1960; Mehl et al. 1964a; Hamel and Moe 1964; Sixth People's Hospital Shanghai 1964; Hayhurst et al. 1974; Harashina and Buncke 1975; Stock et al. 1976; Usui et al. 1978; Hicks et al. 1980; Eisenhard et al. 1980; Tsai et al. 1982; Kessler et al. 1984). The beneficial effects of dry cooling are decreased oxygen demand, a slowdown in oxygen-dependent metabolism and glycolysis, a reduction in reactive hyperemia, and avoidance of venular leakage (Shehadi et al. 1961; Hoffmann 1969; Haff et al. 1975; Grega et al. 1980; Veicsteinas and Comande 1981; Irving and Noakes 1985). As early as 1938, Allen accurately showed that dry cooling of ischemic hind limbs led to a vast reduction in mortality during the reperfusion phase. Similar experiences of reduced postischemic local damage and fewer systemic complications in man have been reported by the Sixth People's Hospital in Shanghai (1975). Successful replantation of a major limb has been reported following even 36 h of *uninterrupted* dry cooling of the extremity. Most victims of amputation, however, cannot be promptly treated due to operational difficulties, nor can their limbs be immediately stored hypothermically. For this reason, particular attention must be paid to limbs that have undergone a warm ischemic period of more than 3 h. Statistically viewed, this is the prevailing situation in most cases of major human limb replantation (McNeil and Wilson 1970; Sixth People's Hospital Shanghai 1975; Morrison et al. 1977; Ferreira et al. 1978; Russel et al. 1984; Maurer et al. 1986). Animal experiments must therefore also include warm ischemic periods of no less than 3 h to produce relevant findings (Steinau et al. 1979).

Quite the same can be said for preischemic flushing-out of severed limbs (Tsai et al. 1982; Rosen et al. 1985; Muramatsu et al. 1985). Few pathophysiological data have been obtained on this procedure, and clinically it has no true relevance.

The insertion of temporary intraluminal shunts has even been recommended and clinically employed to provide oxygen and substrate and reduce metabolite washout (Eger et al. 1974; Adar et al. 1980; Nunley et al. 1981; Johansen et al. 1982).

Isolated perfusion of a disjoined limb, however, would provide a much-needed time span sufficient for careful diagnosis of accompanying injuries, proper evaluation of the patient's suitability for major limb replantation, and treatment of concomitant traumatic shock. While all of these activities are taking place, it is essential that the perfusion solution applied to the limb contains not only substrates, but also oxygen (see Sect. 2.5.3). As already explained, procedures carried out with a heart-lung machine have proven to be too costly and inconvenient for this purpose. Therefore, halogenated hydrocarbons of different concentrations were tested. Though these emulsified fluorocarbons proved capable of adequate oxygen transport function and deoxygenation to the tissue (Geyer et al. 1968; Gould et al. 1982), their presence within the body was often associated with pathological alterations within other organs. Experimentation involving the application of this substance brought on dose-dependent changes in the blood picture (Lutz 1981), increases in pulmonary consistency (Grünert et al. 1981), and accelerated connective tissue formation with proliferation within the liver (Hauk et al. 1977; Schneider et al. 1978; Pfannkuch et al. 1981). Complete destruction of the capillary endothelium following long-term perfusion has also been reported (Smith et al. 1985). Finally, the process by which total elimination of fluorocarbons from the body takes place is not yet totally clear. Major emission occurs with respiration, while traces remain stored within the reticular endothelial system (RES) for up to 6 months without significant degradation changes (Pfannkuch and Schnoy 1979; Pfannkuch et al. 1981; Lundsgaard-Hansen 1980). Despite these findings, the substance has already been used in man (Mitsuno et al. 1982). There have been no reports of anaphylactic reaction or acute pathophysiological changes in the 186 patients treated. However, accumulation within the RES was observed. For this reason the American Food and Drug Administration has refused to release this drug for controlled clinical trial.

The same fluorocarbon substance was employed by Tauber et al. (1981) only as a washout solution in experiments involving the replantation of rabbit hind limbs. They reported accelerated energy-rich phosphate resynthesis following 30 min of perfusion to ischemic limbs that had previously undergone 4-h hypothermic storage. Similar protective mechanisms within ischemic muscle were observed by Schindler et al. (1981) following 8 h of perfusion. A direct contradiction to these findings, however, was reported by Smith et al. in 1985. In portions of amputated human extremities he discovered drops in the levels of energy-rich phosphagens. A study by Karbowski in 1983 produced correlating data. Within the venous efflux he found elevated levels of the cellular enzymes CPK and LDH as well as a drop in pH, despite a continuous supply of fluorocarbons and maintenance of the pO_2 level above 500 mm Hg.

The disadvantages and risks related to halogenated fluorocarbons clearly outweigh the benefits as far as human limb replantation is concerned. As long as the problem of buildup within the RES remains unsolved, the substances should not be employed even as washout/perfusion solutions, as they will leave certain residua within ischemically damaged tissues (see Sect. 3.2.6).

The alternative oxygen and substrate carrier used in our experimental procedures was a stroma-free, oxygenated HbPP solution originally synthesized from erythrocytes in outdated human blood for use as a full blood replacement (Kramlova et al. 1976; Endrich et al. 1976). Unfortunately, this solution has shown itself to possess a limited intravasal staying capacity (Messmer et al. 1978; Bonhard 1982). Along with this, administration in high doses results in disruption of normal kidney function, possibly attributable to small amounts of stroma residuum (Burk et al. 1975). It has also been suggested that changes in intrarenal flow distribution with a decrease in renal plasma flow (Brandt et al. 1951; Savitsky et al. 1978; Stone et al. 1979; Ohshiro et al. 1980), as well as intravasal coagulation disorders (Bucher 1982), could be the responsible factors. A third opinion on the issue has been expressed by Ohshiro et al. (1980), who maintained that obstruction of the renal tubular system results in a direct toxic effect. Histological studies correlating with these clinical observations have shown renal tubular cell necrosis, reabsorbed hemoglobin within tubular cells, hemoglobin cylinder formations within the lumina (Schneider et al. 1976; Unseld et al. 1976; Förster et al. 1977), and hemoglobin deposits within the renal cortex (Andersen et al. 1966).

All of these described pathological changes, however, are strictly dose dependent. In studies carried out on dwarf pigs, Unseld et al. (1976) were able to detect no significant changes, despite plasma levels of 2–3 g%. Primates have exhibited similar results even when 25 ml/kg body wt. of a 6.4% solution was administered, or 25% of total body volume was replaced (Birndorf and Lopas 1970; Savitsky et al. 1978). The infusion of 8–30 g hemoglobin or 250 ml of a 6.4% solution into human volunteer subjects led to a short-term decrease in both urine output and endogenous creatinine clearance as well as to a slightly prolonged thromboplastin time. Normal levels were reestablished 6–10 h later, with absolutely no evidence of change up to 6 months following the experiment.

The elimination of free hemoglobin is achieved through natural degradation pathways with a link to haptoglobin. This complex is absorbed into the RES (mainly liver and bone marrow), where it is later degraded (Keene and Jandl 1965; Andersen et al. 1966). When the normal transport capacity of 128 ± 25 mg/100 ml plasma is overloaded, the excess hemoglobin is excreted via the urine (Devenuto et al. 1979; Birkit et al. 1980). Correlative findings have been published by Bucher (1982), showing values of 100 mg Hb/100 ml blood in cases of intravasal hemolysis. Renal Hb clearance can be calculated at 5 ml plasma/min (Bucher 1982). Still smaller amounts of hemoglobin will be eliminated by cross-linkage of a disassociated molecule to hemopexin, resulting in subsequent breakdown within the liver (Devenuto et al. 1979; Bucher 1982). In case of unexpectedly high levels of free hemoglobin within the blood, the introduction of a haptoglobin solution to the circulation can safely eliminate the burden (Yoshioka et al. 1985).

The same Hb solution used in our rat and canine models has been tried in experimental liver and intestinal perfusions as well as in animal and human openheart procedures for myocardial protection (Förster et al. 1977; Elert and Ottermann 1979). Results demonstrated that the solution possessed an adequate oxygen transport capacity and delivered sufficient oxygen to the tissue (p 50 at a pH of 7.4:27–30 mm/Hg). Employment of this Hb solution in exchange transfusions produced similar positive effects proven by pO_2 measurements on skeletal muscle surfaces (Sunder-Plassman et al. 1973; Messmer et al. 1978). Reviews of the possible uses of such a stroma-free Hb solution were published by Devenuto et al. in 1979 and Dudziak and Bonhard in 1980.

Due to the obviously beneficial effects attributed to the administration of an Hb solution in myocardial cells, this same substance was used experimentally in the amputated extremities of rats and dogs, as well as in traumatically disjoined or amputated tumor-bearing human limbs (Steinau et al. 1979, 1982, 1984; Hild 1983). Perfusion with such a hemoglobin solution can be safely undertaken only when residual hemoglobin levels flushed out from the extremity into the circulatory system do not exceed previously described maximal tolerance plasma concentrations. For this reason, canine hind limbs were rinsed with 200 ml Ringer's solution prior to restoration of autogenous circulation in our experiments.

Clinically, the use of a hemoglobin solution for perfusion provides several advantages:

1. The HbPP solution obtained from outdated whole blood can be easily synthesized in more than adequate quantities (Segal et al. 1981). In the United States alone during 1972 the erythrocytes from 2.7 million pints of donated blood were thrown away, simply because they had become outdated (Abel 1982).
2. Employment of an oxygenated solution (that can be stored for up to 8–9 months) provides simpler operational conditions for replantation centers.
3. The HbPP solution possesses excellent rheological characteristics due to the fact that it contains no cell bodies that could possibly obstruct circulatory passage within the ischemically damaged extremity – relative kinetic viscosity, 1.3; mean mol wt., 65 000 (Cokelet and Meisman 1968).
4. The absence of thrombocytes and erythrocytes within the perfusion medium obviously hinders fatal thrombus formation within the venous portion of the capillary bed (Eriksson 1972; Eriksson et al. 1983).
5. The isosmotic and iso-oncotic solution causes no additional damage to the endothelium and no perfusion-induced edema (O'Connell et al. 1974).

To test the efficiency of perfusion with an oxygenated HbPP solution during the ischemic interval, it was necessary to include certain considerations into the experiment program. It was imperative that the duration of ischemia and the perioperative treatment induce severe morphological changes within the hind limb musculature as well as marked circulatory and metabolic dysfunctions. Therefore, conditions similar to those observed in clinical cases were created. All three experiment groups experienced an initial 3-h ischemic interval at room temperature (22° C). The subsequent 3 h of dry cooling or HbPP perfusion led to an overall ischemic time of 6 h, which has been proven to exceed the ischemic tolerance levels of skeletal muscle (Brückner et al. 1971; Enger 1977). In order that we might observe postischemic morphological changes, the animals were not allowed to die as a result of operational trauma or postoperative postischemia syndrome (Onji et al. 1963; Eiken 1964b; Paul et al. 1965; Brückner et al. 1971). Treatment trials performed prior to the actual experiment yielded valuable information about the necessary infusion of Ringer's lactate, bicarbonate, and Gelifundol (oxypolyge-latine with buffer capacity).

Through the use of a neurovascular pedicle-graft hind-limb model, it was pos-sible to produce isolated ischemic insult to skeletal muscle. Neither perfusion via the endosteal or periosteal vessels nor pressure lesion to the nerves resulted in any irregularities (Thompson et al. 1959; Zucman 1960; Scully et al. 1961; Shehadi et al. 1961; Stalker et al. 1973; Rorabeck 1980).

To reduce postoperative incapacity of movement in the experimental canine models, an early, functionally stable osteosynthesis at the level of the mid femoral shaft was performed. In addition, extensor function within the knee joint was re-established through preservation of the median portion of the extensor muscle with subsequent rejoining to the patellar ligament.

5.3 Metabolic Studies

In an attempt to clarify whether perfusion with an oxygenated HbPP solution during an ischemic interval actually guarantees adequate skeletal muscle metab-olism, levels of the cellular energy-rich phosphagens ATP and CP and of lactate were measured. In contrast to determination of local O_2-pressures with platinum electrodes (Sunder-Plassmann et al. 1973; Messmer et al. 1978; Ehrly 1981), this method directly demonstrates oxygen utilization and energy production within the ischemically damaged cells during the reperfusion phase (Elert and Otter-mann 1979).

Despite the usual occurrence of reactive hyperemia as well as an up to ten fold increase in flow rate within an ischemically damaged and denervated rejoined ex-tremity, a low-flow procedure was employed. Low flow rates of 5 ml/100 g tissue/min were chosen for use, based on the experiments carried out by Stalker et al. (1973), Strohfeld (1973), Chen et al. (1976), and Henrich and Johnson (1978). Following short-term ischemic phases, reactive hyperemia is able to resolve the oxygen debt. However, following long-term periods of ischemia, reactive hy-peremia is mainly responsible for the development of destructive edema (reperfu-sion injury) (Stock 1974; Diana and Laughlin 1974; Little and Reynolds 1976).

Our initial studies, carried out using an oxygenated hemoglobin solution in rat hind-limb models, were compared with the dry-cooling method at 4° C, which at present is the only procedure that has provided any protection to skeletal muscle during the ischemic phase (Sixth People's Hospital Shanghai 1975; O'Brien 1977; Yoshizu et al. 1978; Zwank et al. 1980a; Biemer and Duspiva 1982). Both groups showed significant drops of ATP concentrations to values of 4.9 µmol/g wet tissue weight (Figs. 3, 4). Correlated to this event, CP levels were reduced as well, by approximately 70%, to a value of 4.9 µmol/g wet tissue weight. Perfusion with an oxygenated hemoglobin solution renews the process of energy-rich phosphate synthesis. Peak ATP levels of 7.4 µmol/g wet tissue weight were reached in the 5th h of the experiment, while in the 6th h ATP levels dropped to 6.6 µmol/g wet tissue weight. In contrast to these observations, the curve for the dry-cooling group showed a continuous decrease in the intracellular concentrations of the energy-rich phosphates ATP – 2.4 µmol/g wet tissue weight – and CP – 1.4 µmol/g wet tissue weight. Accordingly, intracellular lactate levels ran an initially parallel course in both groups, after increasing to a mean value of 21 µmol/g wet tissue weight after 2 h at 22° C. However, when perfusion was initiated the curves diverged. Due partly to anaerobic metabolism and partly to impeded washout of acidic waste products, intracellular lactate levels for the dry cooling group climbed to peak values of 32.2 µmol/g wet tissue weight (5th h and 34.1 µmol/g wet tissue weight (6th h). Curves for the perfusion group however, remained at a plateau of 20 µmol/g wet tissue weight during the entire procedure. The statistically significant difference between the two treatment groups ($P < 0.01$) (Table 1) clearly shows the protective effect of perfusion with an oxygenated HbPP solution on ischemically insulted skeletal musculature in rat models.

To imitate typical clinical conditions and circumstances, an initial ischemic interval of 2 h at 22° C was introduced to the experimental procedure. During this time period, the observed drops in energy-rich phosphate levels corresponded with those already reported in the literature following hind-limb tourniquet or amputation procedures in rodents. Levels of energy-rich phosphates showed a parallel course, despite differences within the absolute values caused by variations in method (luciferin/luciferase or enzyme-optical), ischemic interval, species, and dominant muscle fiber type (Bollmann and Flock 1944; Harmann 1949; Threlfall and Stoner 1957; Kauffmann and Albuquerque 1970; Maeiwa et al. 1970; Karlsson 1971; Bohn 1974; Bockmann et al. 1975; Molzberger et al. 1977; Swartz 1978; Jennische et al. 1979). In contrast to the techniques of stop-freezing and/or enzyme-optical testing used by these investigators, the recently introduced nuclear magnetic-resonance technique provides evidence of differing absolute levels and depletion curves within human muscle cells (Thulborn 1981; Newmann 1984; Ostermann 1984). At present, however, interpretation of the data from this technique is difficult; absolute concentration measurements with differentiation of ATP, ADP, AMP, and CP, linked to an intracellular steady-state system, are necessary (Bollmann and Flock 1944; Harmann 1949; Threlfall and Stoner 1957; Kauffmann and Albuquerque 1970; Maeiwa et al. 1970; Karlsson 1971; Bohn 1974; Bockmann et al. 1975; Molzberger et al. 1977; Swartz 1978; Jennische et al. 1979).

As initially mentioned, low-flow perfusion (5 ml/100 g wet tissue/min) during the reperfusion phase will not lead to immediate restitution of energy-rich phosphates. The restoration of autogeneous circulation is much more effective following a 2-h hind-limb tourniquet ischemic period (Bohn 1974). Investigation into intracellular lactate levels produced parallel findings. Bohn also found a marked drop in intracellular lactate concentrations as early as 30 min following restoration of autogenous perfusion. Normal values were observed 2 h later. Low-flow perfusion, however, caused lactate levels to plateau at approximately 21 µmol/g wet tissue weight. These persistently high lactate levels correlate with the findings of Hild (1983), who used oxygenated hemodiluted blood as a perfusion solution in canine hind limbs at a flow rate of 12 ml/100 g tissue wet weight. In 1976, O'Donovan et al. published similar results from experiments with amputated human tumor-bearing limbs. At a flow rate of 5–10 ml/100 g wet tissue weight/min (full blood) they discovered persistently elevated lactate levels as well as rising energy-rich phosphagen values.

The results of these experiments clearly demonstrate the disadvantages of a low-flow perfusion method. However, experience has shown that following ischemic time spans of more than 3 h, the destructive influences of reactive hyperemia can be better avoided through the implementation of low flow rates; the clinically recommended preservation method for amputated limbs of dry cooling at 4° C has proved inferior with reference to energy production.

Further investigations should show whether slight increases in perfusion flow rates following ischemic periods of more than 3 h actually facilitate a quicker return to normal energy-rich phosphagen values without inducing edema-dependent pathological changes within the terminal vascular bed.

5.3.1 Reperfusion Effect

The reperfusion of severed limbs with autogenous circulation often leads to immediate disturbances in systemic metabolism, clotting, and cardiac function. Recognized parameters of the severity of the reperfusion effect (declamping phenomenon, Winninger 1973) are a rapid drop in mean arterial pressure (MAP), increased heart frequency, rising arterial systemic potassium values, and falling arterial pH levels. The degree of ischemic lesion correlates directly to the duration of these alterations (von Saar 1913; Solonen et al. 1968; Brückner et al. 1972; Stock 1974; Dell et al. 1980). Along with these systemic disorders, decreased oxygen and substrate supply and intracellular accumulation of waste products during the ischemic period are responsible for secondary damage. Only after cell organelles have regenerated can resupplied oxygen and substrate once again be efficiently utilized (Deuticke and Gerlach 1966; Kohama et al. 1971; Stock 1974; Trump et al. 1976; Swartz et al. 1978; Jennische et al. 1982).

The factors essentially responsible for primary and secondary damage to the cellular metabolic systems are interstitial and intracellular edema brought on by lactate accumulation and reactive hyperemia. Along with these conditions, released mediators and depletion of energy resources cause membrane permeability disorders and early thrombus formation within the postcapillary vascular bed (Moore et al. 1951; Fairchild et al. 1966; Eriksson et al. 1972; Diana and Laughlin 1974; Little and Reynolds 1976; Hellstrand et al. 1977; Hargens et al. 1981; Muramatsu et al. 1985) (see Sect. 2.5.4).

During the operation and the initial 3 h of storage at room temperature (22° C), the three treatment groups (dry-cooling, HbPP, and sham) exhibited no differences in pH, MAP, or heart frequency. At the 6th h of the procedure mean pH values were found to be between 7.256 and 7.282 (spontaneous respiration) (Fig. 8). Immediately following declamping of the femoral artery and vein, arterial pH levels in blood circulating within the abdominal aorta dropped to a mean of approximately 7.190 and remained there for 1 h. Kußmaul's compensatory respiration phenomenon was observed during this period.

In the HbPP perfusion group, however, stable mean pH values of 7.27–7.283 were recorded, while the sham group exhibited levels of 7.317–7.301 in samples acquired at the same times.

Parallel to these changes during the initial phase of reperfusion, MAP and heart-frequency curves developed courses with intersecting tendencies (Fig. 9). While within the dry-cooling group the MAP dropped sharply from 108 mm Hg to a sustained level of 77 mm Hg following declamping, levels within the sham and HbPP groups remained stable at 108–113 mm Hg. At experiment hours 7 and 8, the dry-cooling group showed MAP levels between 94–97 mm Hg.

A similar trend was seen with reference to heart frequency in that, once again, the dry-cooling group developed an acute increase in heart rate from an average of 108 to 124–130 bpm. Interestingly, in the HbPP and sham groups heart rates showed only slight declines (Fig. 10).

Statistical analysis showed significant differences between the HbPP and dry-cooling groups of $P < 0.01$ for pH and heart frequency and $P < 0.05$ for MAP (Table 2).

Randomly collected samples for the analysis of pO_2, pCO_2, base excess, and bicarbonate also showed tendencies similar to those for the pH. The dry-cooling group exhibited a combined metabolic and respiratory acidosis, while the sham and HbPP groups remained unaffected (Fig. 11).

To clearly demonstrate the significant role of the washout effect during the reperfusion phase, gas analysis of the venous efflux of the isolated extremities was undertaken. After ischemic periods of 2–3 h, rat and canine hind limbs already showed marked acidosis, while pO_2 and pCO_2 curves ran intersecting courses. Following initial pCO_2 values between 83 and 87 mm Hg, the level dropped during perfusion with HbPP to approximately 35–36 mm Hg at the 2nd h. In marked contrast, pO_2 measurement exhibited initial mean values of 35 mm Hg (rat) and 37 mm Hg (dog), climbing to mean venous O_2 levels of 62 mm Hg (dog) and 98 mm Hg (rat) after 2 h of perfusion with HbPP. Measurements of pH, base excess, and bicarbonate also correlated with the data already obtained. At the onset of perfusion there was marked acidosis within the venous efflux (pH 6.9, bicarbonate 11.9, base excess 18.05); this evolved gradually with the low-flow technique to mean values of 7.2 (pH), 16.98 (bicarbonate), and 9.6 (base excess) following 3 h of perfusion in the canine models.

Two further parameters were used to evaluate the quality of the washout effect with an HbPP perfusion model: potassium in the venous efflux (rat) and inorganic phosphate (dog). According to experimental results published by van den Meer et al. (1966), Brückner et al. (1971), and Stock (1974), absolute levels and amounts of potassium within the venous efflux directly correlate with the degree of ischemia-induced damage to muscle cell membrane. Moreover, the massive washout of potassium from ischemically damaged limbs has been identified as a main cause of death with postischemia syndrome (Kristen et al. 1970; Stock 1974).

Ischemia-induced cellular lesions following 3-h storage at a room temperature of 22° C were evident after 10 min of reperfusion within the venous efflux. Mean potassium concentration dropped from an initial 10.8 mEq/l to 8.37 mval/l (30 min) and 6.49 mval/l (1 h). During subsequent hours potassium concentrations between 6.61 and 6.74 ml/l were found (Fig. 6).

Similar results were uncovered by Meroney (1955), Onji et al. (1963), Imai et al. (1964), Fuller et al. (1976), and Pausescu et al. (1976) in connection with Pi

concentrations within the venous efflux. From studies with canine models correlating data can be reported. After 3-h storage at room temperature and subsequent storage at 4° C, there was an identical washout effect during the reperfusion phase (Fig. 11), with Pi concentrations rising to mean values of 7.32 ng/ml
(1 h) and 8.47 ng/ml (2 h) within arterial blood samples. In the HbPP perfusion
group, however, mean values reached only 7.168 ng/ml (1 h) and 7.30 ng/ml (2 h),
while the sham operation group remained basically unchanged, with slightly de-
creasing values of 6.95 ng/ml (1 h) and 6.63 ng/ml (2 h). Interestingly, in all three
groups, initial phosphate concentrations were elevated at a mean of 7.26 ng/ml
(6 h) due to severe amputation trauma.

Data collected from rat and canine limb perfusion studies indicate that despite
the cytoprotective effect that perfusion with an oxygenated HbPP solution provides, complete restitution of the cellular subunits cannot be expected to result
as well. Further investigation into the transmembrane potential of the skeletal
muscle during the reperfusion phase may well provide more insight into its regen-
erative process. Nevertheless, both perfused skeletal muscle and the primarily unaffected remainder of the body as a whole have shown clear benefits.

It is an established fact that elevated potassium levels within the exiting venous efflux are directly responsible for death in experimental and clinical situations. Therefore, the initial washout of potassium from the terminal vascular bed
and the cytoprotective effect provided by HbPP perfusion are very important
(Koslowski 1959; Lapchinsky 1960; Letac et al. 1963; Stock 1974).

The significant differences in MAP and heart frequency among the three experiment groups lead to the conclusion that limb perfusion with an oxygenating
medium prevents destructive reactive hyperemia through early tonicization of the
terminal vascular bed. This preventive mechanism is essentially dependent upon
an adequate level of oxygenation (Fairchild et al. 1966; Barcroft 1972; Hellstrand
et al. 1977). Furthermore, systemic acidosis during the reperfusion phase is also
clearly hindered by perfusion of the extremity with an oxygenating medium,
thereby eliminating yet another life-threatening factor of postischemia syndrome.

5.3.2 Determination of Residua

Following long-lasting ischemia it is quite likely that perfusion media will leak
from the intravasal space into the interstitial realm through ischemically damaged
capillary walls. For this reason, residua determination studies were performed using a ^{125}I-labeled HbPP solution. After a 3-h period of ischemia at room temperature (22° C), canine hind limbs were perfused with an HbPP solution possessing
a basic radioactivity of 8571 ± 340 cpm for 3 h. Subsequent to this procedure, the
vascular bed of the amputated hind limbs was once again flushed with a *nonradiolabeled* HbPP solution (flow rate 4 ml/100 g tissue/min). A rapid decrease in
activity was exhibited by an asymptotic descending curve. As early as 10 min into
the nonradiolabeled perfusion procedure, less than 4% of the original radioactive
dose could be detected. This descent continued to a final level of 1% at 16 min
(Fig. 14). Samples taken from skin, subcutaneous tissue, and muscle of the hind

extremities revealed the continued presence of the extravasally stored, radiola-beled HbPP solution (Figs. 16 and 17). Conversion of the radioactive cpm into g HbPP/kg tissue produced readings between 7.21 and 13.25 g HbPP/kg tissue after 3 h of perfusion with the radiolabeled medium. After 1 h of perfusion with the nonlabeled HbPP solution, mean values of 1.0–3.217 g HbPP/kg tissue were measured. Maximally tolerable concentrations of free hemoglobin within the hu-man circulatory system have been discussed previously by Brandt et al. (1951), Savitsky et al. (1978), and Bucher (1982). According to their data, the speed of elimination of free hemoglobin within the efflux of the canine hind limbs and the absolute concentrations of free hemoglobin found within the ischemically dam-aged tissues are not likely to result in overall systemic damage. To assure yet an-other measure of safety, flushing of an amputated extremity for 10 min with Ringer's lactate before declamping has proven to drastically reduce the residual presence of the HbPP solution. In sharp contrast to fluorocarbons, which also leak through ischemically damaged capillary walls and are stored within the tissue of the limb, HbPP molecules follow a safer and more natural course of degrada-tion (see Sect. 3.2.3). Histopathological investigations carried out on canine livers and kidneys at various points following ischemia up to 1.5 years support these conclusions.

5.4 Histomorphological and Electron-Optical Findings

Before perfusion of amputated limbs with any solution is undertaken, the method should be tested to exclude any possible side effects within the microstructures of the capillary bed and muscle cells. In addition, the potential for intensification of the ischemic lesions during the reperfusion phase and the regeneration phase must be carefully considered (Harmann 1949; Rotter 1958, 1959). In an effort to dis-cover whether perfusion with an iso-oncotic and isotonic, stroma-free HbPP so-lution would lead to destructive changes within the endothelial lining and inter-stitial space similar to those reported in the literature with various other solutions (Little et al. 1973; O'Connel et al. 1974; McNamara et al. 1985; Smith et al. 1985; Rosen et al. 1985; Mazer et al. 1986), we performed electron-optical studies of the vascular structures of rat hind limbs. Following 2 h of ischemia at 22° C and sub-sequent 4-h perfusion with HbPP, endothelial linings and capillary lumina showed no pathological changes (Figs. 16 and 17). The surrounding muscle fiber exhibited normal structure, but a slight pericapillary edema due to long-term low-flow perfusion was observed.

In cases of hind limb ischemia of more than 2 h duration, significant progres-sive insult to the muscle fibers and capillary system has been observed, its inten-sity correlated to the species (Mäkitie et al. 1977a; Gordon et al. 1978 – rat models), (Harman 1948; Dahlbäck 1970; Santavirta et al. 1979; Brunelli and Fac-chetti 1981 – rabbit models), (Scully et al. 1961; Stenger et al. 1962; Enger 1977; Stock et al. 1976 – canine models), (Tountas and Bergman 1977; Patterson and Klenerman 1979 – in apes). It is for this reason that the experimental procedures used in our canine studies involved an initial 3-h ischemic period at room temperature, followed by either *3 h dry cooling* or *3 h HbPP perfusion* to guarantee the incidence of significant histomorphological and ultrastructural muscle tissue damage without resulting in death of the animal (Hargens et al. 1981). During the initial reperfusion phase, both treatment groups developed *qualitatively* similar changes. At 24 and 48 h postoperatively, only minor scattered areas of muscle cell necrosis appeared in the HbPP perfusion group; in the dry-cooling group, however, 70%–80% of the muscle fibers exhibited ischemia-induced rhabdomyolysis (Figs. 18, 19, 25, and 26). Cellular lesions within the anterior tibial muscle were markedly more severe than those found within the gastrocnemius musculature (Fuhrmann and Crisman 1959; Hargens et al. 1981). It is believed that increased compartment pressure during the reperfusion and/or the predominance of a specific fiber type (with low ischemic tolerance) is the responsible additional factor in the development of muscle cell necrosis. Ischemia-induced lesions of the intracellular structures have been described in the literature several times (Stenger et al. 1962; Karpati et al. 1974; Stock 1974; Hanzlikova and Schiaffiono 1977; Mäkitie 1977; Heffner and Barron 1978; Tountas and Bergman 1977; Ludatscher et al. 1981; Muramatsu et al. 1985). Other pathological conditions such as expanding edema, vacuolation, degeneration of the sarcoplasmic reticulum, disruption of the myofibrillar structures, clump formations of debris, and reservoirs of edema were observed within the muscle cells of the dry-cooling group (Figs. 29, 30, and 37). Mitochondrial destruction manifested as edematous ballooning, giant mitochondria formation, loss of cristal structure, and the formation of trilaminar structures (Figs. 30, 37, 38). These pathological changes were observed in the HbPP perfusion group as well, but they were not nearly as severe.

Interestingly, during the reperfusion phase in the HbPP group, capillary edema was only slight, while within the dry-cooling group massive interstitial edema and marked stenosis of the capillary lumina developed. These conditions, along with endothelial blistering, subtotal occlusion of the lumina, and loss of organized capillary wall structure with exposition of subendothelial structures and clinging thrombocytes, granulocytes, and erythrocytes, are typically characteristic of the "no-reflow phenomenon" (Figs. 31, 32, and 38) (Strock and Manjo 1969 b; Willms-Kretschmer and Manjo 1969; Fuchs 1970; Eriksson 1972; Eriksson et al. 1983; Fonkalsrud et al. 1976).

By the 5–8th postoperative day, histologically observed invading macrophages removed any fiber fragments present. Simultaneously, surviving myonuclei and/or satellite cells underwent gradual conversion into immature fiber regenerates between or within the sarcolemmal sheath. Parallel to this generation of new fibers connective tissue cells tried to invade/proliferate into the same space (Figs. 19, 20, 26) (Karpati et al. 1974; Adams et al. 1975; Mäkitie 1977; Carlson 1981).

These regenerational attempts were found only focally within the HbPP perfusion group (Fig. 26), while within the dry-cooling group a sharply contrasting disseminating young-fiber pattern appeared as a sign of required fiber revitalization (Fig. 20).

On the 5th postischemic day, electron-optical studies provided evidence that the cristae structure of the mitochondria was already regenerating, even within areas of partial or complete fibrillolysis (Figs. 33, 34, 39).

Tissue specimens collected from the dry-cooling group during 3 months to 1.5 years of follow-up showed permanent major and minor areas of scar tissue development along with scattered aggregations of macrovacuolar metaplastic fatty tissue between the regenerated muscle cells. The fibers exhibited irregular variations in caliber as well as jagged borders (Figs. 23, 24). Ultrastructurally, areas of persistent fibrillolysis were frequently found in fibers that appeared normal histomorphologically (Fig. 35). Along with these findings, bizzare mitochondrial structures were seen in areas of intensified transparency.

The HbPP perfusion group fibers, however, demonstrated totally regular cell structure with homogeneous calibers histologically, in specimens collected up to 1.5 years post ischemia (Figs. 28, 40). Ultrastructurally, the pathological conditions frequently seen in the dry-cooling group were seldom observed in the HbPP perfusion group (Fig. 41).

Whether the appearance of permanently deformed mitochondrial structures can be interpreted as intracellular residuum of ischemic damage remains to be quantitatively clarified. Experiments performed by Tountas and Bergman (1977) have shown evidence of such singular pathological organelle structures even within normal skeletal musculature.

To prove that the chosen method of ischemic insult to the musculature of the neurovascular pedicled hind limb did not result in further coincidently occurring lesions, histological and electron-optical studies were performed within the sham group. At no time following the operation were any pathological changes found within the anterior tibial muscle or the gastrocnemius musculature.

5.5 Conclusions

The histological and electron-optical studies carried out on skeletal musculature clearly confirm the protective effect of low-flow HbPP perfusion as superior to that of the clinically recommended method of dry cooling during the chosen ischemic intervals. Along with marked dimunition of fiber necrosis, HbPP perfusion will help to maintain the capillary wall structure and unobstructed lumina. Under controlled circumstances of induced ischemia parallel to those often found in clinical situations, an accelerated repair rate and *restitutio ad integrum* were observed. This was certainly not the case with the dry-cooling group in which scattered aggregations of scar tissue, fatty metaplasia, and regenerated fibers with jagged borders and varying calibers were seen. The results of ultrastructural studies correlated with the histomorphological findings. Immediately following initial ischemic cell destruction and subsequent regeneration, focal fibrillolysis and unusually formed mitochondrial structures were frequently seen in the dry-cooling group. This was seldom the case with HbPP-treated muscles.

Histological studies of kidney and liver tissue provided differing findings. In the dry-cooling group discrete signs of resolved shock syndrome were detected. The tissues from the HbPP perfusion group showed no such pathological conditions, however. Up to 1.5 years following perfusion treatment no residua from liberated hemoglobin were found.

6 Summary

The replantation of predominantly muscular major limbs has not yet become a routine clinical procedure, as even in highly specialized replantation centers early and late complications of the **postischemia syndrome** remain a potential threat. The possibilities of multiple organ failure (MOF), emergency reamputation, ineffective functional end results (especially in cases of close proximal amputation levels), and death sharply influence a surgeon's decision for amputation or replantation.

Pathophysiological analysis has shown ischemia-induced myopathy and microangiopathy of the skeletal musculature to be responsible for high perioperative morbidity, and the extent of muscle cell necrosis has been found to be directly correlated with deficiencies in functional rehabilitation.

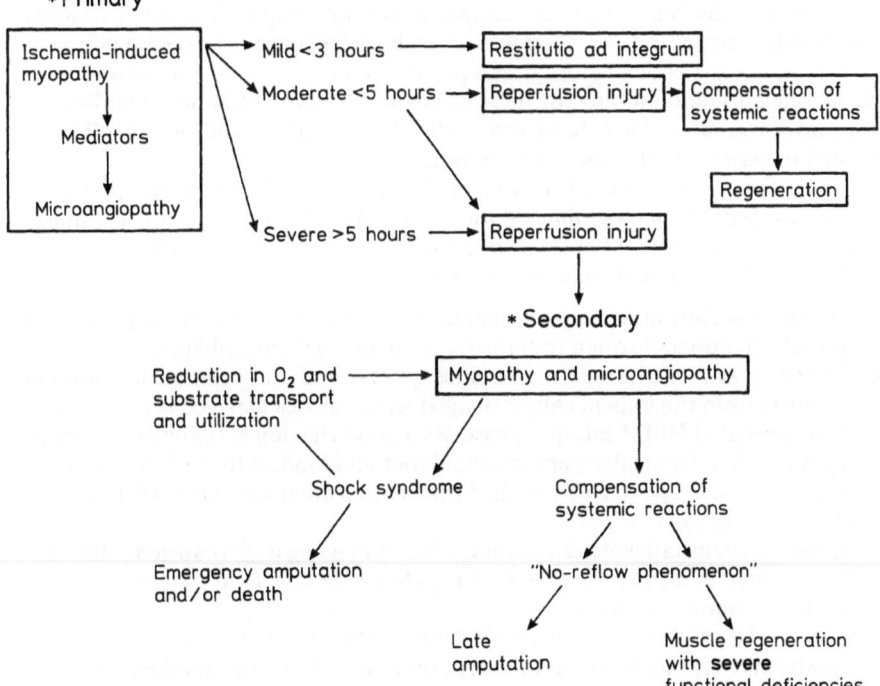

Fig. 42. Postischemia syndrome in major limb replantation

Figure 42 demonstrates schematically the possible pathophysiological pathways of the postischemia syndrome in major limb replantation. Following long periods of ischemia, early thrombus formation and cells clinging to the capillary wall triggered by mediators within the postcapillary venules, and pathological changes of the capillary endothelium, result in initially scattered and finally generalized areas of obstructed perfusion (**no-reflow phenomenon**).

Interestingly, potentially fatal sequalae related to ischemia-induced lesions of the affected extremity can be seen throughout the rest of the body. One such condition is a massive drop in mean arterial pressure due to a decrease in total peripheral resistance parallel to a sharp increase in heart frequency (**declamping phenomenon**). At the same time, the washout of cellular potassium and acid metabolites leads to life-threatening hyperkalemia and severe systemic acidosis. The loss of plasma into the expanding edematous extremity is primarily responsible for volume-deficiency shock, while the influx of lysosomal proteolytic enzymes, collagen, and tissue thromboplastin is likely to cause formation of disseminated microthrombi with renal failure and pulmonary complications (ARDS). Shock, severe systemic acidosis, and marked myoglobinemia bring on characteristic precipitation of "muscle pigment" within the renal tubular system.

Finally, when all of the above acutely threatening complications have been adequately checked and brought under control, the rapid edema-induced pressure jumps within the fascio-osseous compartments are responsible for secondary muscle cell necrosis and potential loss of the limb (**compartment syndrome**).

Numerous methods of storage and perfusion have been tried to provide prophylaxis against and therapy for these local and systemic mechanisms of destruction; however, some have been too costly, too complex, and/or not effective enough to earn general clinical acceptance.

In contrast to previously tested methods reported in the literature, perfusion with an oxygenated hemoglobin solution (HbPP) clearly provides the advantage of a constant O_2 delivery system during the interval of limb separation.

Results of experiments have proven that:

1. Low-flow perfusion with an oxygenated HbPP solution guarantees protection of skeletal muscle through resynthesis of energy-rich phosphagens.
2. Sufficient washout of acid metabolites, potassium, and cellular degradation products from the ischemically damaged terminal vascular bed is provided.
3. An oxygenated HbPP solution possesses a good rheological capacity for passing through ischemically stenosed capillaries and hinders thrombus formation within the postcapillary venous bed (mean molecular weight: 65 000, relative kinematic viscosity: 1.3).
4. Based on quantitative determination of residua using a ^{125}I-labeled HbPP solution, there is no reason to expect negative side effects in potential clinical trials with human subjects.
5. Storage of a previously oxygenated HbPP solution (up to 8 months) is unproblematic and the method of administration is technically uncomplicated.

From a clinical point of view, perfusion with an oxygenated HbPP solution would achieve the following conditions and substantially improve the chances for success in major limb replantation:

1. Sufficient time for careful and critical examination of the patient and adequate time for diagnosis and pretreatment of the frequent concomitant multiple traumas.
2. Preoperative normothermic preparation of the severed limb.
3. Prophylactic treatment for early and late-appearing complications (reperfusion injury, compartment syndrome.
4. Improved functional end results through diminished ischemic muscle cell necrosis and enhanced regeneration potential.
5. Increased in the number of instances of partial replantation for distalization of proximal stumps and/or stump coverage through microvascular free-flaps harvested from the amputated limb.

7 References

Aagard OC (1913) Die Lymphgefäße der Extremitätenmuskeln. Anat Hefte (1) 47:602–620

Abbott WM, Maloney RD, Mclabe CC, Lee ChE, Wirthlin LS (1982) Arterial embolism: a 44-year perspective. Am J Surg 143:460–464

Abel WG (1982) Blood substitute oxygen carriers. NY State J Med 82:1429–1433

Adams RD, Denny-Brown D, Pearson CM (1975) Diseases of muscle, 2nd edn. Harper and Row, New York

Adar R, Schramek A, Khodadi J, Zweig A, Golcman L, Romanoff H (1980) Arterial combat injuries of the upper extremity. J Trauma 20:297–302

Albrektsson T (1982) Ischaemia and bone grafts. Scand J Plast Reconstr Surg 19:21–24

Allbrook DB, Aitken JT (1951) Reinnervation of striated muscle after acute ischemia. J Anat 85:376–394

Allen FM (1938) Resistance of peripheral tissues to asphyxia at various temperatures. Surg Gynecol Obstet 67:746–751

Aloisi M, Mussini J, Schiaffino S (1973) Activation of muscle nuclei in denervation and hypertrophy. In: Kakulas BA (ed) Basic research in myology. Excerpta Medica, Amsterdam

Amelang E, Prasad CM, Raymond RM, Grega GJ (1981) Interactions among inflammatory mediators on edema formation in the canine forelimb. Circ Res 49:298–306

Ames A, Wright RL, Kowada M, Thurston JM, Majno G (1968) Cerebral ischemia II, the no-reflow phenomenon. Am J Pathol 52:437–447

Amundson B, Haljamäe H (1976) Skeletal muscle metabolites as possible indicators of imminent death in acute hemorrhage. Eur Surg Res 8:311–320

Anderl H (1977) Storage of a free groin flap. Chir Plast 4:41–43

Andersen MN, Mouritzen OV, Gabrielli ER (1966) Mechanisms of plasma hemoglobin clearance after acute hemolysis in dogs. Ann Surg 164:905–912

Angliss VE (1974) Upper-limb-deficient children. Am J Occup Ther 28(7):407–414

Ängquist KA, Sjöström M (1981) Skeletal muscle ischemia: fine structural changes in different muscle fibres after intermittent peripheral arterial insufficiency compared with clinical physiological data. Bibl Anat 20:566–571

Appelgren L (1972) Perfusion and diffusion in shock. Acta Physiol Scand [Suppl] 378:5–72

Appell HJ (1984) Zur Variabilität des Kapillarmusters im Skelettmuskel unter Berücksichtigung der Faserverteilung. In: Hammersen F (ed) Die Mikrozirkulation des Skelettmuskels. Karger, Basel

Arango A, Illner H, Shires GT (1976) Role of ischemia in the induction of changes in cell membrane during hemorrhagic shock. J Surg Res 20:473–476

Armbrustmacher VM (1978) Skeletal muscle in denervation. Pathol Annu 2:1–33

Artigue RS, Hyman WA (1976) The effect of myoglobin on the oxygen concentration in skeletal muscle subjected to ischemia. Ann Biomed Eng 4:128–137

Ashton H (1962) Critical closing pressure in human peripheral vascular beds. Clin Sci 22:79–87

Ashton H (1975) The effect of increased tissue pressure on blood flow. Clin Orthop 113:15–26

Aub JC (1944) A toxic factor in experimental traumatic shock. N Engl J Med 231:71–75

Aub JC, Brues AM, Kety SS, Nathanson TT, Nutt AL, Pope A, Zamecnik PC (1945) The toxic factors in experimental traumatic shock. IV. The effects of the intravenous injection of the effusion from ischemic muscle. J Clin Invest 24:845–849

Babior BM (1978) Oxygen-dependent microbial killing by phagocytes. N Engl J Med 298I:659–668

Bagge U, Amundson B, Braide M (1981) A method to observe and quantitate leucocyte interference with flow in in the skeletal muscle microcirculation. Bibl Anat 20:557–560

Barcroft H (1972) An enquiry into the nature of the mediator of the vasodilatation in skeletal muscle in exercise and during circulatory arrest. J Physiol 222:P99–118

Bardenheuer B (1911) Die Entstehung und Behandlung der ischämischen Muskelkontraktur und Gangrän. Dtsch Z Chir 108:44–201

Barnard RJ, Edgerton R, Furnkawa T, Peter JB (1971) Histochemical, biochemical and contractile properties of red, white and intermediate fibres. Am J Physiol 220:410–414

Bar-Or O, Dotan R, Inbar O, Rothstein A, Karlsson J, Tesch P (1980) Anaerobic capacity and muscle fiber-type distribution in man. Int J Sports Med 1:82–85

Bartlett RA (1986) The effect of superoxide dismutase on macromolecular leakage and leucocyte accumulation in the skin microcirculation after ischemia and reperfusion. 31st Plast Res Council ASPRS, Norfolk.

Baudet J (1981) Major limb replantation: panel discussion. 6th Symposium of the International Society for Reconstructive Microsurgery, Melbourne, 1981

Baue AE, Chandry JH, Wurth MA, Sayeed MA (1974) Cellular alterations with shock and ischemia. Angiology 25:31–42

Baumgartner R (1973) Beinamputation und Prothesenversorgung bei arteriellen Durchblutungsstörungen. Enke, Stuttgart

Baumgartner R (1977) Amputation und Prothesenversorgung beim Kind. Enke, Stuttgart

Baumgartner R (1981) Management of bilateral upper-limb amputees. Orthop Clin North Am 12(4):971–976

Bayliss WM (1919) Further observation on the results of muscle injury and their treatments. National Health and Medical Research Committee, London, special report, series 26:23–26

Beasley RS (1981) General considerations in managing upper-limb amputations. Orthop Clin North Am 12(4):743–749

Benner KU, Gaehtgens P, Schickendantz S (1975) Hemodynamic and functional consequences of intravascular platelet aggregation in skeletal muscle. Microvasc Res 9:310–316

Bereiter-Hahn J (1974) Auswirkung von O_2-Mangel auf Gefäßendothelzellen. In: Breddin K (ed) Trasylol Symposium, Frankfurt. Schattauer, Stuttgart, 1975, pp 205–215

Berger A (1983) Replantationschirurgie – Indikation und Grenzen. Hefte Unfallheilkd 162:144–157

Berger A (1984) Replantation surgery, indications and limitations. In: Tscherne H (ed) Fractures with soft tissue injury. Springer, Berlin Heidelberg New York

Berger A, Kolacny M, Passl R, Piza H (1980) Die Replantation ganzer Extremitäten – Pro und Contra. Hefte Unfallheilkd 148:557–564

Berggren A, Weiland AJ, Dorfman H (1982) The effect of prolonged ischemia time on osteocyte and osteoblast survival in composite bone grafts revascularised by microvascular anastomoses. Plast Rec Surg 69:290–298

Bergmeyer HU (1963) Methods of enzymatic analysis. Academic, New York

Betz EH (1966) Relation of the regenerated muscle fibers to the connective tissue. Int Res Cytol 19:218–220

Biemer E (1977) Replantation von Fingern und Extremitätenteilen. Chirurg 48:353–359

Biemer E (1983) Limb replantation: panel discussion. 7th symposium International Society for Reconstructive Surgery, New York

Biemer E (1984) Reconstruction of the hand with two-toe en-bloc transfer and neurovascular flaps from the foot. In: symposium on clinical frontiers in reconstructive microsurgery. Mosby, St. Louis

Biemer E, Duspiva W (1982) Reconstructive microvascular surgery. Springer, Berlin Heidelberg New York

Biglioli P, Santa A, Ferozzi G, Bandera A, Clerici U (1973) Renal function after revascularisation. J Cardiovasc Surg 14:578–585

Birkit HG, Heinrich P, Brandstätter W, Fritzsche L (1980) Zur Verwendung stromafreier Hämoglobinlösung als Blutersatz. Z Exp Chir 13:230–234

Birndorf NJ, Lopas H (1970) Effect of red cell stroma-free hemoglobin solution on renal function in monkeys. J Appl Physiol 29:573–578

Blachar J, Fong JSC, Chadarevian JP, Drummond KN (1981) Muscle extract infusion in rabbits, a new experimental model of the crush syndrome. Circ Res 49:114–124

Blaisdell FW, Lim RC, Amberg JR, Choy SH, Hall AD, Thomas AN (1966) Pulmonary microembolism. Arch Surg 93:776–786

Blaisdell FW, Steele M, Allen RE (1978) Management of acute lower extremity arterial ischemia due to embolism and thrombosis. Surgery 84:822–834

Blalock A (1930) Experimental shock: the cause of the low blood pressure produced by muscle injury. Arch Surg 20:959–996

Blechschmidt E (1932) Die Architektur des Fersenpolsters. Verh Anat Ges 41:20–68

Blomfield LB (1945) Intramuscular vascular patterns in man. Proc R Soc Med 38:617–618

Bockmann EL, Berne RM, Rubino R (1975) Release of adenosine and lack of release of ATP from contracting skeletal muscle. Pflugers Arch 355:229–241

Bohn HJ (1974) Status energiereicher Phosphate und glykolytischer Metabolite in der Extremitätenmuskulatur der Ratte bei Ischämie und in der postischämischen Erholung. Inaugurat dissertation, University of Cologne

Bollmann JL, Flock EV (1944) Changes in phosphate of muscle during tourniquet shock. Am J Physiol 142:290–297

Bond RF, Manley ES, Green HD (1967) Cutaneous and skeletal muscle vascular responses to hemorrhage and irreversible shock. Am J Physiol 212I:488–497

Bondy SC, Purdy J, Carroli JE, Kaiser K (1976) The rate of nutrient supply to normal and denervated slow and fast muscle, and its relation to muscle blood flow. Exp Neurol 51:678–683

Bonhard K (1976) Sauerstoff transportierende Therapeutika aus abgelaufenem Konservenblut. Proceedings of congress in blood transfusion and immunology. Biotest Institute, Frankfurt

Bonhard K (1982) Which is the foreseeable clinical application of oxygen-carrying blood substitutes (fluorocarbons and hemoglobin solutions?) Vox Sang 42:97–109

Booth FW, Kelso JR (1973) Effect of hind-limb immobilisation on contractile and histochemical properties of skeletal muscle. Pflugers Arch 342:231–238

Bradley WG, Thomas PK (1974) Neuropathies due to vascular disease – Ischemic neuropathy. In: Walton J (ed) Disorders of the voluntary muscle. Churchill Livingstone, London

Brandt JL, Frank R, Lichman HC (1951) The effect of hemoglobin solutions on renal functions in man. Blood 6:1152–1158

Breitenfelder J (1982) Das Amputationsfolge-Spätsyndrom aus orthopädischer Sicht – Ergebnisse einer Nachuntersuchung von 108 OS-Amputierten. Z Orthop 120:611

Brettschneider H (1964) Über die Innervation der Muskelgefäße. In: Bad Oeynhäuser Gespräche, vol 6. Springer, Berlin Göttingen Heidelberg, pp 37–56

Brooke MH (1973) Muscle fiber typing. In: Kalkulas BA (ed) Basic research in myology. Excerpta Medica, Amsterdam

Brooke MH, Kaiser KK (1980) The use and abuse of muscle histochemistry. Ann NY Acad Sci 228:121–144

Brooks B (1922) Pathologic changes in muscle as a result of disturbances of circulation. Arch Surg 5:188–216

Brown M, Cotter M, Hudlicka O, Smith M, Urbova G (1973) Metabolic changes in long-term stimulated fast muscles. In: Howald H (ed) Proceedings of the international symposium on biochemistry of exercise, Magglingen, 1973

Brown PW (1981) The rational selection of treatment for upper-extremity amputations. Orthop Clin North Am 12(4):843–848

Brückner UB, Schmier J (1974) Beeinflussung der postischämischen Veränderungen in der Hinterextremität im Tierversuch. In: Breddin K (ed) Trasylol symposium. Schattauer, Stuttgart

Brückner UB, Hermann H, Schmier J, Stenger E, Ulmer HE (1971) Hämodynamische Veränderungen im Tourniquet-Schock des Hundes. Z Kreislaufforsch 60:740–751

Brückner UB, Opherk D, Schmier J, Treumer H, Schwarz G (1972) Kreislaufdynamik und Kontraktilität des Herzens im Tourniquet-Schock des Hundes bei Hemmung der Blutgerinnung und der Xanthinoxydase. Z Kreislaufforsch 61:161–178

Brues AM, Cohn WE, Kety SS, Nathanson TT, Nutt AL, Tibbets DM, Zamecnik PC, Aub JC (1945) The toxic factors in experimental traumatic shock. II. Studies on electrolyte and water balance in shock. J Clin Invest 24:835–838

Brunelli G, Facchetti F (1981) Anatomical and histological alterations induced by warm and cold ischemia. In: Brunelli G (ed) Ischemia and reimplantation. Liviana, Padua

Bucher U (1982) Klinik und Therapie des hämolytischen Transfusionszwischenfalls. Umweltmedizin 2:29–34

Buchtal F, Kamieniecka Z, Schmalbruch H (1974) Fibre types in normal and diseased human muscle and their physiological correlates. In: Milhorat AT (ed) Exploratory concepts in muscular dystrophy. II. Excerpta Medica, Amsterdam

Buck-Gramcko D (1974) Ischämische Kontrakturen an Unterarm und Hand. Handchirurgie 6:141–158

Bütikofer E, Mollegres J (1968) Akute ischämische Muskelnekrosen, reversible Muskelverkalkungen und sekundäre Hypercalcämie bei akuter Anurie. Schweiz Med Wochenschr 26:961–965

Bundesanstalt für Arbeit (1981/82) Zugänge von Rehabilitanden. Amtliche Nachrichten No 10, No 11 (1982)

Bundschuh HD, Suchenwirth R, Davis W (1973) Histochemical changes in disuse atrophy of human skeletal muscle. In: Kakulas BA (ed) Basic research in myology. Excerpta Medica, Amsterdam

Burck HC, Eichner G, Sedleczek T (1975) Das akute Nierenversagen nach Hämoglobin-Infusion mit und ohne Erythrozytenstromata am Kaninchen. Res Exp Med 166:79–94

Buri P (1973) Traumatologie der Blutgefäße. Huber, Bern

Burke RE (1974) The correlation of physiological properties with histochemical characteristics in single muscle units. Ann NY Acad Sci 228:145–159

Burkhardt K, Stankovic P (1973) Die leucozytäre Phagozytose im Schock. Langenbecks Arch Chir [Suppl]:347–349

Burnstock G, Griffith SG (1983) Die Innervation der glatten Muskulatur terminaler Gefässe. In: Messmer K (ed) Vasomotion und quantitative Kapillaroskopie. Karger, Basel

Bywaters EGL (1944) Ischemic muscle necrosis. JAMA 124:1103–1109

Cain SM, Chapler CK (1980) O_2 extraction by canine hind limb during alpha-adrenergic blockade and hypoxic hypoxia. J Appl Physiol 48:630–635

Cannon MB, Bayliss WM (1919) Note on muscle injury in relation to shock. National Health Medical Research Committee, London, special report, series 26:19–23

Carlson BM (1973) The regeneration of skeletal muscle – a review. Am J Anat 137:119–149

Carlson BM (1981) The biology of muscle transplantation. In: Freilinger G (ed) Muscle transplantation. Springer, Vienna New York

Carlson BM, Hansen-Smith FM, Magon DK (1979) The life history of a free muscle graft. In: Mauro A (ed) Muscle regeneration. Raven, New York

Carrel A, Guthrie C (1906) Complete amputation of the thigh with replantation. Am J Med Sci 131:297–301

Carroll D (1965) A quantitative test of upper-extremity function. J Chronic Dis 18:479–491

Castaigne P, Cathala HP, Mastropailo C, Dry J, Gras E (1966) Les réponses des nerfs et des muscles à des stimulations électriques au cours d'une épreuve de garrot ischémique chez l'homme normal. Rev Fr Etud Clin Biol 11(4):373–387

Castle ME, Reyman TA (1984) The effect of tenotomy and tendon transfers on muscle fiber types in the dog. Clin orthop 186:302–310

Chachques JC, Mitz V, Vernejoul P, Daillet G, Fontanliran F, Vilain R (1983) Etude expérimentale de la circulation lymphatique après réimplantation de membres. Ann Chir Plast Esthet 28:195–198

Chaiklin H, Warfield M (1973) Stigma management and amputee rehabilitation. Rehabil Lit 34(69):162–172

Chait LA, May JW, McO'Brien B, Hurley JW (1978) The effects of the perfusion of various solutions on the no-reflow phenomenon in experimental free flaps. Plast Rec Surg 61:421–430

Chambers R, Zweifach BW, Lowenstein BE (1944) The peripheral circulation during the tourniquet shock syndrome in the rat. Ann Surg 120:791–802

Chan PH, Schmidley JW, Fishman RA, Longar SM (1984) Brain injury, edema and vascular permeability changes induced by oxygen-free radicals. Neurology 34:315–320

Chandler JG, Knapp RW (1967) Early definitive treatment of vascular injuries in the Vietnam conflict. JAMA 202:960–966

Chang JB (1981) Successful replantation of upper arm. Vasc Surg 15:163–180

Chase RA (1970) The severely injured upper limb: to amputate or reconstruct: that is the question. Arch Surg 100:382–287

Chaudry JH, Sayeed MM, Baue AE (1976) Alternations in high-energy phosphates in hemorrhagic shock as related to tissue and organ function. Surgery 79:666–668

Chen ChW (1981) Major limb replantation, Panel discussion. 6th Symposium of the International Society for reconstructive Microsurgery, Melbourne, 1981

Chen HJ, Goodman AH, Granger HJ (1976) Mechanisms of increased tissue oxygen delivery following release of arterial occlusion in canine skeletal muscle and skin. Adv Exp Med Biol NY 75:667–674

Chen ChW, Yun-Quing Q, Zhong-Jia Yu (1978) Extremity replantation. World J Surg 2:513–524

Chen ChW, Meyer VE, Kleinert HE, Beasley RW (1981) Recent indications and contraindications for replantation as reflected by long-term functional results. Orthop Clin 12:849–870

Chen ChW, Yang DJ, Chang DS, Chao YL (1982) Microsurgery. Springer, Berlin Heidelberg New York

Chernov MS (1973) Limb replantation. JAMA 224:528

Cherry GW, Ryan TJ (1976) The effect of ischemia and reperfusion on tissue survival. In: Ryan TC (ed) Microvascular injury. Saunders, London

Chishueit'an Hospital Peking (1975) Replantation of severed limbs. Chin Med J 1(4):265–274

Chiu DH, Wang HWA, Blumenthal MR (1976) Creatine phosphokinase release as a measure of tourniquets' effect on skeletal muscle. Arch Surg 111:71–74

Chou SM, Nonaka J (1977) Satellite cells and muscle regeneration in diseased human skeletal muscle. J Neurol Sci 34:134–145

Christeas N, Balas P, Giannikas A (1969) Replantation of amputated extremities. Am J Surg 118:68–74

Chung Shan Medical College, Kwangchow (1973) Replantation of severed limbs. Chin Med J 6:70–73

Clawson D, Seddon HJ (1960a) The result of repair of the sciatic nerve. J Bone Joint Surg 42B:205–212

Clawson DK, Seddon HJ (1960b) The late consequences of sciatic nerve injury. J Bone Joint Surg 42B:213–225

Clothiaux P, Wood MB, Vanhoutte PM (1985) Effective ischemia on bone vasomotor reactivity. 8th Symposium of the International Society for Reconstructive Microsurgery, Paris, 1985

Clyne CAC, Weller RO, Bradley WG, Silber DI, O'Donnel TF, Callow AD (1982) Ultrastructural and capillary adaptation of gastrocnemius muscle to occlusive peripheral vascular disease. Surgery 92:434–440

Cokelet GR, Meiseman HJ (1968) Rheological comparison of hemoglobin solutions and erythrocyte suspensions. Science 162:275–277

Collan Y, Alho A (1973) Ultrastructure of the kidneys in tourniquet shock. Eur Surg Res 5:333–347

Collins GM (1969) Kidney preservation for transportation. Lancet 2:1219–1222

Colmers F (1909) Über die durch das Erdbeben in Messina am 28. Dezember 1908 verursachten Verletzungen. Arch Klin Chir 90:701–729

Colmers F (1920) Die Verschüttungsverletzung des Krieges. Ergeb Chir Orthop 12:670–677

Conner AN (1911) Prolonged external pressure as a cause of ischemic contracture. J Bone Joint Surg 53B:118–122

Constance TJ (1955) An experimental study of the reaction of skeletal muscle to injury. Aust J Exp Biol 33:257–274

Coonrad RW, Milford LW (1981) Results of microsurgery in orthopedics: the committee on the upper extremity. Educ Semin Am Acad Orthop Surg 665

Cormier JM, Devin R (1969) Traitement des oblitérations arterielles aigües des membres. 71st congress of surgery, Association française de chirurgie, Paris

Cormier JM, Legrain M (1962) L'hyperkaliémie, complication gravissime des syndrome d'ischemie aigüe des membres. J Chir 83:473–483

Cunningham JN, Chires GT, Wagner J (1971) Cellular transport defects in hemorrhagic shock. Surgery 70:215–222

Dahlbäck LO (1970) Effects of temporary tourniquet ischemia on striated muscle fibres and motor end-plates. Scand J Plast Rec Surg [Suppl]:7–87

Dahn J, Lassen NA, Westling H (1967) Blood flow in human muscle during external pressure or venous stasis. Clin Sci 32:467–473

Danese C, Howard JM, Bower R (1962) Regeneration of lymphatic vessels: a radiographic study. Ann Surg 156:61–67

Davies EJ, Fritz BR, Clippinger FW (1970) Amputees and their prostheses. Artificial Limbs 14:19–48

Dederich R (1982) Wiederherstellungs-chirurgische Maßnahmen – Plastisch-chirurgische Maßnahmen an Oberschenkel- und Unterschenkelstümpfen. Z Orthop 120:613–614

Dell PC, Seaber AV, Urbaniak JR (1980) The effect of systemic acidosis on perfusion of replanted extremities. J Hand Surg 5:433–442

Dellon AL, Jabaley ME (1982) Reeducation of sensation in the hand following nerve suture. Clin Orthop 163:75–79

Del Maestro RF, Thaw HH, Björk J, Planke M, Arfors KE (1980) Free radicals as mediators of tissue injury. Acta Physiol Scand [Suppl] 492:43–57

Delorme TL, Shaw RS, Austen WG (1964) A method studying "normal" function in the amputated human limb using perfusion. J Bone Joint Surg 46A:161–164

Denck H, Russe O, Hold M (1977) Mißerfolge durch verspätete Operationen bei Gefäßverletzungen. Wien Med Wochenschr 127:740–741

Denotter G (1968) The clinical problems encountered in replantation of limbs. Arch Chir Neerl 20:127–139

Denzler G, Stürz H, Tönnis D, Walcher K (1973) Muskelveränderungen bei Kaninchen nach Kniegelenksversteifung. Arch Orth Unfall Chir 77:165–180

Dery R (1965) Metabolic changes induced in the limb during tourniquet ischemia. J Can Anesth Soc 12:367–378

Deuticke B, Gerlach E (1966) Abbau freier Nucleotide in Herz, Skelettmuskel, Gehirn und Leber der Ratte bei Sauerstoffmangel. Pflugers Arch 292:239–254

De Venuto E, Friedman HJ, Neville JR, Peck CC (1979) Appraisal of hemoglobin solution as a blood substitute. Surg Gynecol Obstet 149:417–436

Diana JN, Laughlin MH (1974) Effect of ischemia on capillary pressure and equivalent pore radius in capillaries of the isolated dog hind limb. Circ Res 35:77–101

Dias PLR, Simpson JA (1974) Effects of cross-innervation on the motor end-plates of fast- and slow-twitch muscles of the rabbit. Q J Exp Phys 59:213–223

Dobson JG, Rubio R, Berne RM (1971) Role of adenine nucleotides, adenosine, and inorganic phosphate in the regulation of skeletal muscle blood flow. Circ Res 29:375–384

Doi K, Kawai S, Kotani H, Kuwata N (1983) Multiple organ failure after revascularisation of lower limb. 7th Symposium of the International Society of Reconstructive Microsurgery, New York

Donski PK, Franklin JD, Hurley JV, McO'Brien B (1980) The effect of cooling on experimental free flap survival. Br J Plast Surg 33:353–360

Donski PK, Fischer F, Meyer VE (1984) Beitrag zur Häufigkeit und Bedeutung von Epiphysen- und epiphysen-nahen Verletzungen bei Replantationen im Bereich der oberen Extremität bei Kindern. Handchir Mikrochir Plast Chir 16:196–200

Dorman JD (1973) The histopathology of neurogenic muscular atrophy. In: Pearson CM (ed) The striated muscle. Williams and Wilkins, Baltimore

Dudziak R, Bonhard K (1980) The development of hemoglobin preparations for various indications. Anaesthesist 29:181–189

Duncan GW, Blalock A (1942) The uniform production of experimental shock by crush injury: possible relationship to clinical crush syndrome. Ann Surg 115:684–697

Duran WN (1979) Microcirculatory hemodynamics. In: Serafin D (ed) Microsurgical composite tissue transplantation. Mosby, St. Louis

Duran WN, Marsicano TH (1979) Anatomy of the microcirculation. In: Serafin D (ed) Microsurgical composite tissue transplantation. Mosby, St. Louis

Dyckerhoff H, Schörcher F (1938/39) Über die Beziehungen zwischen den „Frühgiften" und den Komponenten des Blutgerinnungssystems. Biochem Z 300:193–197

Dyckerhoff H, Schörcher F, Torres J (1938/39) Über die Darstellung einer toxischen Substanz (Myotoxin) aus frischem Muskelgewebe. Biochem Z 300:197–203

Edfeldt H, Thomson D (1980) Early hemodynamic and respiratory changes following tourniquet release – influence of large doses of methylprednisolone. Acta Chir Scand [Suppl] 499:45–55

Echtermeyer V (1985) Das Kompartmentsyndrom. Hefte Unfallheilkd 169

Eger M, Schmidt B, Török G, Khodadadi J, Goldmann L (1974) Replantation of upper extremities. Am J Surg 128:447–450

Ehrlich W (1965/66) Zur Verwendung des Kunstarms im gewerblichen Leben. Verh Dtsch Orthop Ges 52:357–358

Ehrly AM (1981) Messungen des Gewebesauerstoffdrucks im ischämischen Muskelgewebe von Patienten mit arteriellen Verschlusskrankheiten mittels Mikro-Platin-Stichelektroden. In: Ehrly AM (ed) Messung des Gewebesauerstoffdrucks bei Patienten. Witzstrock, Baden-Baden

Eigler FW (1974) Das Tourniquet-Syndrom – Pathophysiologie und Klinik. In: Breddin K (ed) Neue Aspekte der Trasylol Therapie. Schattauer, Stuttgart

Eiken O (1964a) Limb replantation: technique and immediate results. Arch Surg 88:48–54

Eiken O (1964b) Limb replantation: the pathophysiological effects. Arch Surg 88:54–66

Eiken O, Mayer RF, Nabseth DC, Apostolou K, Deterling RA (1964) Limb replantation: long-term evaluation. Arch Surg 88:66–77

Eis G (1956) Die Legende vom abgeschnittenen Pferdebein. Tierärztl Umschau 11:152–154

Eisenberg BR (1974) Quantitative ultrastructural analysis of adult mammalian skeletal muscle fibres. In: Milhorat HT (ed) Exploratory concepts in muscular dystrophy. Excerpta Medica, Amsterdam

Eisenhardt HJ, Prangenberg G, Isselhard W, Pichlmaier H, Klein PJ (1980) Studies of energy metabolism in ischemic skeletal muscle of the rat in different procedures of storing and conservation. Thorc Cardiovasc Surg 28:35–36

Elert O, Ottermann U (1979) Cardioplegic hemoglobin perfusion. A method of providing optimal myocardial protection. J Thorac Cardiovasc Surg 27:245–247

Elert O, Steinau HU, Schneider M (1982) Beeinflussung des postischämischen Kompartmentsyndroms durch Hämoglobinperfusion. Langenbecks Arch Chir 358:504

Ellsworth ML, Goldfarb RD, Alexander RS, Bell DR, Powers SR (1981) Microembolization-induced oxygen utilization impairment in the canine gracilis muscle. Adv Shock Res 5:89–99

Ely JF (1977) Lower forearm replantation. In: Daniel RK (ed) Reconstructive microsurgery. Little Brown, Boston

Endrich B, Jesch F, Peters W, Meßmer K (1976) Reanimation nach akutem Blutverlust mit stromafreier Hämoglobinlösung. Langenbecks Arch Chir [Suppl]:54–57

Enerson DM (1966) Cellular swelling I, II. Arch Surg 163:169–174, 537–544

Engber WD (1971) Replantation of extremities. Surgery 132:901–916

Engel AG, Stonnington HA (1980) Morphological effects of denervation of muscle. A quantitative ultrastructural study. Ann NY Acad Sci 228:68–88

Engel WK, Hawley RJ (1977) Focal lesions of muscles in peripheral vascular disease. J Neurol 215:161–168

Enger EA (1977) Cellular metabolic response to regional hypotension and complete ischemia in surgery. Acta Chir Scand [Suppl] 481

Erbslöh F (1972) Sekundäre Muskelveränderungen bei peripheren Nervenläsionen. Med Mitt 46:59–83

Eriksson E (1972) Microcirculation in skeletal muscle in cat. Elander, Gothenburg

Eriksson E, Anerson WA, Reploge RL (1974) Effects of prolonged ischemia on muscle microcirculation in the cat. Surg Forum 25:254–255

Eriksson E, Reploge RL, Glagov S (1987) Reperfusion of skeletal muscle after ischemia. (to be published)

Fabiani JN, Joseph D, Carpentier A (1976) Ischémie temporaire et phénomène de non-réperfusion. Lettre d'information, 6 GAM

Fairchild HM, Ross J, Guyton AC (1966) Failure of recovery from reactive hyperemia in the absence of oxygen. Am J Physiol 210:490–492

Farber JL, Chien KR, Mittnacht S (1981) The pathogenesis of irreversible cell injury in ischemia. Am J Pathol 102:271–281

Faulkner JA, Maxwell LC, White TP, Niemeyer JH (1979) Characteristics of autografted mammalian skeletal muscles. In: Mauro A (ed) Muscle regeneration. Raven Press, New York

Feng LJ (1986) Release of arachidonic acid metabolites and prostaglandins in the no-reflow phenomenon of replanted rat hind limb. 31st Plastic Research Council, American Society for Plastic and Reconstructive Surgery, Norfolk

Ferreira MC, Marques EF, Azze RJ (1978) Limb replantation. Clin Plast Surg 5:211–221

Fichtner G (1968) Das verpflanzte Mohrenbein. Zur Interpretation der Kosmas und Damian Legende. Med Hist J 3:87–98

Fisher StV, Gullickson G (1978) Energy cost of ambulation in health and disability: a literature review. Arch Phys Med Rehabil 59:124–133

Flohe L, Loschen G (1984) Sauerstoffradikale als Entzündungsmediatoren. In: Biochemie und Klinik der Superoxid-Dismutase. Perimed, Erlangen

Florin I, Gerhards F, Knapp TW, Fuhrmann J, Stürmer R (1981) Psychologische, medizinische, demographische und rehabilitative Variablen in ihrer Beziehung zum Rehabilitationserfolg bei einseitig beinamputierten Männern. Research report FL 117/1 of the Deutsche Forschungsgemeinschaft, Marburg

Förster H, Hoos J, Schneider M, Hauck H (1977) Zur Verwendung von stromafreien Hämoglobinlösungen als Blutersatz. Infusionstherapie 4:122–126

Folkow B (1964) Autoregulation in muscle and skin. Circ Res 14 [Suppl 1.2]:119–124

Fonkalsrud EW, Sanchez M, Zerubauel R, Lassaletta L, Smeesters C, Mahoney A (1976) Arterial endothelial changes after ischemia and perfusion. Surg Gynecol Obstet 142[II]:715–721

Fontijne WPJ, Mook PH, Elstrodt JM, Wildevuur CRH (1985) Effects of acute bleeding on oxygen supply to the skeletal muscle in dog. Eur Surg Res 17:61–68

Frank GR (1972) Limb replantation. In: Aitken GT (ed) The child with an acquired amputation. Natl Acad Sci, Washington

Frankenthal L (1916) Über Verschüttungen. Virchows Arch 222:332–345

Freeman BA, Crapo JD (1982) Biology of disease. Free radicals and tissue injury. Lab Invest 47:412–426

Friedmann LW (1978) The surgical rehabilitation of the amputee. Thomas, Springfield

Fronek K, Zweifach BW (1975) Microvascular pressure distribution in skeletal muscle and the effect of vasodilatation. Am J Physiol 228:791–796

Fuchs U (1970) Postischämische Permeabilitäts- und Perfusionsstörungen im Skelettmuskel. Acta Biol Med Germ 25:193–195

Fuchs U, Bodendieck P (1975) Postischemic circulation disturbances. Z Mikroskop Anat Forsch 89:49–62

Fuhrmann FA, Crismon JM (1959) Early changes in distribution of sodium, potassium and water in rabbit muscle following release of tourniquets. Am J Physiol 166:424–432

Fuller TJ, Carter NW, Barcenas C, Knochel JP (1976) Reversible changes of the muscle cell in experimental phosphorus deficiency. J Clin Invest 57[II]:1019–1024

Furnas DW (1970) Growth and development in replanted forelimbs. Plast Rec Surg 46:445–453

Fürst P, Bergström J, Hultman E, Vinnars E (1976) Intermediary energy metabolism for the catabolic state with special regard to muscle tissue. In: Wilkinson AW (ed) Metabolism and the response to injury. Pitman, Kent

Furuse A, Brawley RK, Struve E, Gott VL (1973) Skeletal muscle gas tension: indicator of cardiac output und peripheral tissue perfusion. Surgery 74:214–222

Gaehtgens P, Benner KU, Schickedanz S (1976) Nutritive and non-nutritive blood flow in canine skeletal muscle after partial microembolisation. Pflugers Arch 361:183–189

Gaudio E, Pannarale L, Marinozzi G (1984) A tridimensional study of microcirculation in skeletal muscle. Vasc Surg 11/12:372–381

Gebert G, Schnitzer W, Piechowiak H, Nguyen-Duong H, Schiebe M (1974) Mechanismus der Ödembildung in Skelettmuskulatur nach Ischämie. In: Breddin K (ed) Neue Aspekte der Trasyloltherapie. Schattauer, Stuttgart

Gelberman RH, Garfin SR, Hergenröder PT, Mubarak SJ, Menon J (1981) Compartment syndromes of the forearm. Clin Orthop 161:252–261

Gerdin B, Arfors KE, Schoenberg M (1985) Die pathophysiologische Bedeutung freier Sauerstoffradikale. In: Messmer K (ed) Angiodynamik und Angiopathie. Zuckschwerdt, Munich

Gergely J (1974) Biochemical aspects of muscular structure and function. In: Walton JN (ed) Disorders of the voluntary muscle. Churchill Livingstone, London

Geyer RP, Monroe RG, Taylor K (1968) Survival of rats totally perfused with a fluorocarbon-detergent preparation. In: Norman JC (1968) Organ perfusion and preservation. Appleton Century Crofts, New York

Ghussen F, Stock W (1979) Die Wirkung von Methylprednisolon auf den Verlauf des experimentellen Tourniquet-Schocks des Hundes. Res Exp Med 176:87–95

Gibson T (1965) Early free grafting: the restitution of parts completely separated from the body. Br J Plast Surg 18:1–11

Gidlöf A, Hammersen F, Larsson J, Lewis DH, Liljedahl SO (1979) Endothelial swelling and impairment of reflow in human skeletal muscle capillaries provoked by prolonged tourniquet ischemia. Acta Chir Scand [Suppl] 493; 490–494

Gidlöf A, Larsson J, Lewis DH, Hammersen F (1981) Capillary endothelial alterations affecting reperfusion after ischemia in human skeletal muscle. Bibl Anat 20:572–577

Gollnick PD, Sjödin BS, Karlsson J, Jansson E, Saltin B (1974) Human soleus muscle: a comparison of fibre composition and enzyme activities with other leg muscles. Pflugers Arch 348:247–255

Gordon L, Buncke HJ, Townsend JJ (1978) Histological changes in skeletal muscle after temporary occlusion of arterial and venous supply. Plast Reconstr Surg 61:576–580

Gould SA, Rosen AL, Sehgal LR, Sehgal HL, Rice CL, Moss GS (1982) Red cell substitutes: hemoglobin solution or fluorocarbon. J Trauma 22:736–740

Graf P, Duspiva W, Geißendörfer K, Schmeller ML (1984) Der Einfluß von variablen Anoxämiezeiten auf das Knochenlängenwachstum. Unfallheilkunde 87:251–255

Graf P (1984) Untersuchungen über das Längenwachstum juveniler Meerschweinchentibias nach variierenden Anoxämiezeiten. Dissertation, Technical University, Munich

Granger DN, Rutili G, McCord JM (1981) Superoxide radicals in feline intestinal ischemia. Gastroenterology 81:22–29

Gray SD, Renkin EM (1978) Microvascular supply in relation to fibre metabolic type in mixed skeletal muscles of rabbits. Microvas Res 16:406–425

Green HN, Stoner HB (1952) Muscle ischemia and the reaction to injury with special reference to the role of nucleotides. In: Le muscle: etude de pathologie et biologie. L'expansion Scientifique Française, Paris

Grega GJ, Maciejko JJ, Raymond RM, Sak DP (1980) The interrelationship among histamine, various vasoactive substances and macromolecular permeability in the canine forelimb. Circ Res 46:264–275

Griffith D (1960) cited in: Hardy EG, Tibbs DJ (eds) Acute ischemia in limb injuries. Br Med J 1:1001–1005

Groom AC, Ellis CG, Potter RF (1984) Die Architektur und Erythrozytenperfusion der Endstrombahnen im Skelettmuskel und deren Veränderungen während der Kontraktion. In: Hammersen F (ed) Die Mikrozirkulation des Skelettmuskels. Karger, Basel

Gross EM (1978) Autopsy findings in drug addicts. Pathol Annu 2

Grünert A, Hirlinger WK, Herrmann (1981) Tierexperimentelle Erfahrungen mit Fluosol. International Symposium on oxygen-carrying colloidal substitutes, Mainz, 1981

Grunewald WA, Sowa W (1977) Capillary structure and O_2 supply to tissue. Rev Physiol Biochem Pharmacol 77:150–209

Guth L, Yellin H (1971) The dynamic nature of the so-called fiber types of mammalian skeletal muscles. Exp Neurol 31:277–300

Guthrie C (1912) Blood vessel surgery and its applications. Arnold, London

Gutschi S, Koter H, Pascher O, Koch G (1981) Zur Problematik der Spät-Revaskularisation nach Gefäßverletzung. Angiology 3:317–320

Hackradt A (1917) Über akute tödliche vasomotorische Nephrosen nach Verschüttung. Dissertation, University of Munich

Haddy FJ, Scott JB (1968) Metabolically linked vasoactive chemicals in local regulation of blood flow. Phys Rev 48:688–707

Haff RC, Klebanoff G, Brown BG, Koreski WR (1975) Asanguineous hypothermic perfusion as a means of the total organism preservation. J Surg Res 19:13–19

Hagberg S, Haljamäe H, Röckert H (1970) Shock reactions in skeletal muscle. Acta Chir Scand 136:23–28

Haimovici H (1973) Myopathic-nephrotic-metabolic syndrome associated with massive acute arterial occlusion. J Cardiovasc Surg 14:589–600

Haimovici H (1979) Muscular, renal, and metabolic complications of acute arterial occlusion: myonephropathic-metabolic syndrome. Surgery 85:461–468

Hales R, Pullen D (1982) Hypotension and bleeding diathesis following attempted arm replantation. Anaesth Intensiv 10:359–361

Haljamäe H, Enger E (1975) Human skeletal muscle energy metabolism during and after complete tourniquet ischemia. Ann Surg 182:9–14

Hall RH (1944) Whole upper-extremity transplant for human beings: general plans of procedure and operative technique. Ann Surg 119:12–23

Hall-Craggs ECB (1978) Ischemic muscle as a model of regeneration. Exp Neurol 60:393–399

Hallenbeck JM (1977) Prevention of postischemic impairment of microvascular perfusion. Neurology 27:3–10

Halmagyi AF, Baker CB, Campbell HN, Evans JG, Mahoney CJ (1969) Replantation of a completely severed arm followed by reamputation because of failure of innervation. Can J Surg 12:222–228

Halpern AA, Nagel DA (1980) Anterior compartment pressure in patients with tibial fractures. J Trauma 20:782–790

Halsted WS (1922) Replantation of entire limbs without suture of vessels. Proc Natl Acad Sci USA 8:181–186

Hamel AL, Moe JH (1964) Effect of total ischemia on hind limbs of dogs subjected to hypothermia. Surgery 55:274–280

Hammersen F (1965) Zum Feinbau der Muskelkapillaren in abgeschnürten Extremitäten der Ratte. Anat Anz 115:367–375

Hammersen F (1970) The terminal vascular bed in skeletal muscle with special regard to the problem of shunts. In: Crone C (ed) AB-Foundation, symposium II. Munksgaard, Copenhagen

Hammersen F (1971) Anatomie der terminalen Strombahn. Urban & Schwarzenberg, Munich

Hammersen F, Hammersen E (1985) Das Endothel – ein disseminiertes metabolisch aktives Organ. In: Messmer K (ed) Angiodynamik und Angiopathie. Zuckschwerdt, Munich

Hanson KM (1964) Autoregulation in the hind limb. Circ Res 14:125–129

Hanzlikova V, Schiaffino S (1977) Mitochondrial changes in ischemic skeletal muscle. J Ultrastruct Res 60:121–133

Harashina T, Buncke H (1975) Study of washout solutions for microvascular replantation and transplantation. Plast Rec Surg 56:542–548

Hardy EG, Tibbs DJ (1960) Acute ischemia in limb injuries. Br Med J 1:1001–1005

Hargens AR, Akeson WH, Mubarak SJ, Owen CA, Evans KL (1978) Fluid balance within the canine anterolateral compartment. J Bone Joint Surg 60A:499–505

Hargens AR, Gershuni DH, Gould RN, Gelbermann RH, Zweifach SS, Mubarak SJ, Akeson WH (1981) Tissue necrosis associated with tourniquet ischemia. Bibl Anat 20:599–601

Harman JW (1948) The significance of local vascular phenomena in the production of ischemic muscle necrosis in skeletal muscle. Am J Pathol 24:142:625–641

Harman JW (1949) The recovery of skeletal muscle fibres from acute ischemia as determined by histological and chemical methods. Am J Pathol 25 II:741–754

Harriman DGF (1977) Ischemia of peripheral nerve and muscle. J Clin Pathol [Suppl 30] 11:94–104

Harris WH, Malt RA (1974) Late results of human limb replantation. J Trauma 14:44–52

Hassler O (1970) The angioarchitecture of normal and denervated muscle. Neurology 20:1161–1164

Hauk H, Schneider M, Hofmann H, Voss J, Förster H, Hübner K (1977) Experimentelle Untersuchungen an der Ratte zur Leber- und Milzvergrößerung nach Gabe synthetischer Sauerstoffträger (Fluorkohlenwasserstoffe). Verh Dtsch Ges Pathol 61:357

Hayhurst JW, McO'Brien B, Ishida H, Baxter TJ (1974) Experimental digital replantation after prolonged cooling. Hand 6:134–141

Heffner RR, Barron SA (1978) The early effects of ischemia upon skeletal muscle mitochondria. J Neurol Sci 38:295–315

Heger H, Millstein S, Hunter GA (1985) Electrically powered prosthesis for the adult with upper limb amputation. J Bone Joint Surg 67B:278–281

Hellstrand P, Johansson B, Norberg K (1977) Mechanical, electrical, and biochemical effects of hypoxia and substrate removal on spontaneously active vascular smooth muscle. Acta Phys Scand 100:69–83

Hendley ED, Schiller AA (1954) Change in capillary permeability during hypoxemic perfusion of rat hindleg. Am J Physiol 179:216–220

Henneman E, Olson CB (1965) Relation between structure and function in the design of skeletal muscle. J Neurophysiol 28:581–598

Henrich H, Johnson PC (1978) Influence of arterial pressure on reactive hyperemia in skeletal muscle capillaries. Am J Physiol 234:H352–360

Hentz VR (1981) Successful replantation of a totally avulsed scalp following ischemia. Ann Plast Surg 7:145–148

Heugel E, Molzberger H, Isselhard W (1973) Ödementwicklung und Erholung des Muskelstoffwechsels nach einseitiger Extremitätenischämie der Ratte nach Anwendung des Proteinaseninhibitors Trasylol. Langenbecks Arch Chir [Suppl]:17–20

Hewitt RL, Frazier DM, Drapanas T (1971) Reactive edema and necrosis after restoration of blood flow in the limb. J Surg Res 11:248–253

Hicks TE, Boswick JA, Solomons CC (1980) The effect of perfusion on an amputated extremity. J Trauma 8/20:632–648

Hild P (1983) Tierexperimentelle Untersuchungen zur Eignung von Blutersatzstoffen als alleinige Sauerstoffträger im extrakorporalen Kreislauf am Modell der isolierten Extremitätenperfusion. Habilitationsschrift University of Giessen

Hirsch H, Gaehtgens P (1965) Entstehung von Thrombozytenaggregaten durch Extremitätenischämie beim Hund. Z Gesamte Exp Med 139:227–237

Höpfner E (1903) Über Gefäßnaht, Gefäßtransplantationen und Replantationen von amputierten Extremitäten. Arch Klin Chir 70:417–471

Hörl M, Hörl WH (1985) Effect of tourniquet ischemia on carbohydrate metabolism of dog skeletal muscle. Eur Surg Res 17:53–60

Hörl M, Hörl WH, Heidland A (1982) Proteinkatabolismus und Tourniquetschock: Rolle der proteolytischen Enzyme. Chirurg 53:253–257

Hofmann KT (1969) Zur Pathophysiologie der Extremitätenischämie und des Tourniquetschocks. Ann Univ Sarav 16:1–81

Hofmann CA, Bunch WH, Kestnbaum JS (1981) Management of psychological problems. In: Am Acad Orthop Surg (eds) Atlas of limb prosthesis. Mosby, St. Louis

Hogan EL, Dawson DM, Romanul FCA (1965) Enzymatic changes in denervated muscle. II. Biochemical studies. Arch Neurol 13:274–282

Honig CR (1977) Hypoxia in skeletal muscle at rest and during transition to steady work. Microvasc Res 13:377–398

Hoover RM (1964) Problems and complications of amputees. Clin Orthop 11/12:47–52

Horn JS, Sevitt S (1951) Ischemic necrosis and regeneration of the tibialis anterior muscle after rupture of the popliteal artery. J Bone Joint Surg B 33:348–358

Horn JS (1969) The reattachment of severed extremities. In: Apley AG (ed) Recent advances in orthopedics. Williams and Wilkins, Baltimore

Hudlicka O (1973) Muscle blood flow. Zwets and Zeitlinger, Amsterdam

Hudlicka O, Tyler KR, Wright AJA, Ziada AM (1984) Wachstum und Vermehrung der Kapillaren in der Skelettmuskulatur. In: Hammersen F (ed) Die Mikrozirkulation des Skelettmuskels. Karger, Basel

Hübner K, Zimmermann H (1959) Experimentelle Untersuchungen über den Einfluß der temporären Ischämie auf die Blutbildung. Acta Haematol 22:209–231

Hughes CN (1958) Arterial repair during the Korean War. Ann Surg 147:555–561

Hunter J Sir (1784) Treatise on the blood, inflammation and gunshot wounds. London

Hutton M, Rhodes RG, Chapman G (1982) The lowering of postischemic compartment pressures with mannitol. J Surg Res 32:239–242

Illner H, Shires GT (1980) The effect of hemorrhagic shock on potassium transport in skeletal muscle. Surg Gynecol Obstet 150:17–25

Im MJ, Manson PN, Bulkley GB, Hoopes JE (1985) Effects of superoxide dismutase and allopurinol on the survival of acute island flaps. Ann Surg 201:357–359

Imai S, Riley AL, Berne RM (1964) Effect of ischemia on adenine nucleotides in cardiac and skeletal muscle. Circ Res 15:443–450

Imatami JH, Miller StH, Demuth RJ, Buck DC (1984) Environmental and pharmacologic alterations to ameliorate the no-reflow phenomenon. Surg Forum: 599–601

Inoue T (1967a) Replantation of severed limbs. J Cardiovasc Surg 8:31–39

Inoue T (1967b) Factors necessary for successful replantation of upper extremities. Ann Surg 165:225–238

Irving GA, Noakes TD (1985) The protective role of local hypothermia in tourniquet-induced ischaemia of muscle. J Bone Joint Surg 67-B:297–301

Jacobson SH (1962) Microvascular surgery. Dis Chest 41:220

Jaeger SH, Tsai TM, Kleinert HE (1981) Upper-extremity replantation in children. Orthop Clin North Am 12:897–907

Järhult J, Mellander S (1974) Autoregulation of capillary hydrostatic pressure in skeletal muscle during regional arterial hypo- and hypertension. Acta Physiol Scand 91:32–41

Jaffe DM, Terry RD, Spiro AJ (1978) Disuse atrophy of skeletal muscle. J Neurol Sci 35:189–200

Jansson I, Loven L, Rammer L, Lennquist S (1985) Pulmonary trapping of platelets and fibrin after musculoskeletal trauma. J Trauma 25:288–298

Jasinski B, Brütsch H (1952) Zur Pathogenese, Prognose und Therapie traumatischer Myoglobinurien. Schweiz Med Wochenschr 82:29–33

Jeger E (1912) Die Chirurgie der Blutgefäße und des Herzens. Hirschwald, Berlin (Reproduction: Springer, Berlin Heidelberg New York 1973)

Jennings RB (1976) Relationship of acute ischemia to functional defects and irreversibility. Circulation 53:I26–I29

Jennische E, Amundson B, Haljamäe H (1979) Metabolic response in feline red and white skeletal muscle to shock and ischemia. Acta Physiol Scand 106:39–45

Jennische E, Hagberg H, Haljamäe H (1982) Extracellular potassium concentration and membrane potential in rabbit gastrocnemius muscle during tourniquet ischemia. Pflugers Arch 392:335–339

Jenny G (1980) Psychischer Hospitalismus als Folge posttraumatischer Osteomyelitis. Hefte Unfallheilkd 148:608–612

Jepson PN (1926) Ischemic contracture. Ann Surg 84:785–795

Jianu J (1913) Beiträge zum Studium der Transplantationen. Arch Klin Chir 102:58–61

Jöbsis FF, Boyd JB, Barwick WJ (1979) Metabolic consequences of ischemia and hypoxia. In: Derafin D (ed) Microsurgical composite tissue transplantation. Mosby, St. Louis

Johanson K, Bernstein EF (1979) Revascularisation of the ischemic canine hind limb by arteriovenous reversal. Ann Surg 190:243–253

Johansen K, Bandyk D, Thiele B, Hansen ST (1982) Temporary intraluminal shunts: resolution of a management dilemma in complex vascular injuries. J Trauma 22:395–402

Johnson PC (1977) The myogenic response and the microcirculation. Microvasc Res 13:1–18

Josza L (1976a) Ultrastrukturelle Veränderungen der menschlichen Skelettmuskulatur nach Sehnen- und Nervenverletzungen. I. Feinstrukturelle Abweichungen der Handmuskeln nach Sehnenverletzungen. Arch Orthop Unfall Chir 84:179–186

Josza L (1976b) Ultrastrukturelle Veränderungen der menschlichen Skelettmuskulatur nach Sehnen- und Nervenverletzungen. II. Feinstrukturelle Veränderungen nach Verletzung des motorischen Nerven. Arch Orthop Unfall Chir 84:187–197

Judet R (1962) Cited in: Salesses M, Moussu A, Aupecle M: Jeux observations „princeps" de section traumatique quasi complète du bras. Mem Acad Chir, Paris, 88:930–940

Jupiter JB, Tsai TM, Kleinert HE (1982) Salvage replantation of lower-limb amputation. Plast Rec Surg 69:1–8

Kappus H (1984) Toxizität von Sauerstoffradikalen – Biologische Funktion und schädliche Wirkung auf das Gewebe. In: Biochemie und Klinik der Superoxid-Dismutase. Perimed, Erlangen

Karbowski A, Pennig D, Brug E (1983) Gewebekonservierung vor mikrochirurgischer Versorgung von Gliedmaßenamputationen. 13th Congress of the Union of German Plastic Surgeons, Hanover, 1983.

Karlsson J (1971) Lactate and phosphagen concentrations in working muscle of man. Acta Phys Scand [Suppl] 358

Karlsson J, Willerson JT, Leshin SJ, Mullins CB, Mitchell JH (1975) Skeletal muscle metabolites in patients with cardiogenic shock or severe congestive heart failure. Scand J Lab Invest 35:73–79

Karpati G (1976) Trophic regulation of the structure and function of skeletal muscle. In: Daniller AM (ed) Symposium on microsurgery. Mosby, St. Louis

Karpati G, Engel WK (1968) Correlative histochemical study of skeletal muscle after suprasegmental denervation, peripheral nerve section and skeletal fixation. Neurology 18:681–692

Karpati G, Carpenter S, Melmed C, Eisen AA (1974) Experimental ischemic myopathy. J Neurol Sci 23:129–161

Karpf M, Stock W, Gebert E, Kruse-Jarres JD, Zimmermann W (1973) Stoffwechselveränderungen und Restitution nach temporärer Tourniquet-Ischämie beim Menschen. Langenbecks Arch Chir [Suppl]:307–311

Kaspar U, Wiesmann U, Mumenthaler M (1969) Necrosis and regeneration of the tibialis anterior muscle in rabbit. Histological changes. Arch Neurol 21:363–372

Kaspar U, Mumenthaler M, Steiner A, Ludin HP, Wiesmann (1971) Regeneration of tibialis anterior muscle in rat after complete excision and reimplantation of muscle fragments. Z Neurol 200:18–32

Katzenstein R, Mylon E, Wintermitz MC (1973) The toxicity of thoracic duct fluid after
release of tourniquets. Am J Physiol 139:307–312

Kauffmann FC, Albuquerque EX (1970) Effect of ischemia and denervation on metabolism of fast and slow mammalian muscle. Exp Neurol 28:46–63

Kaufmann T, Hurwitz DJ (1983) Systemic and local oxygen effects on rat axial-pattern flap
survival. Chir Plastica 7:201–209

Kawamura M, Sakakibara K, Jusa T (1978) Effect of increased oxygen on peripheral circulation in acute, temporary limb hypoxia. J Cardiovasc Surg 19:161–168

Keene WR, Jandl JH (1965) The sites of hemoglobin catabolism. Blood 26:705–719

Kennedy TJ, Miller ST, Nellsis SH, Buck D, Flain SF, Graham WP, Davis TS (1981) Effects of transient ischemia on nutritient flow and A-V shunting in canine hind limb.
Ann Surg 193:225–263

Kerrigan CL, Daniel RK (1982) Critical ischemia time and the failing skin flap. Plast Reconstr Surg 69:986–989

Kerrigan CL, Zelt RG, Daniel RK (1984) Secondary critical ischemia time of experimental
skin flaps. Plast Reconstr Surg 74:522–526

Kerstein MD, Zimmer H, Dugdale FE, Lerner E (1977) Successful rehabilitation following
amputation of dominant versus nondominant extremities. Am J Occup Ther 31:313–
315

Kessler ME, Rothaus KO, Goulian D (1984) A model for hypothermic preservation of amputated extremities utilizing continuous perfusion. Surg Forum: 605–607

Kety SS, Nathansson IT, Nutt AL, Pope A, Zamecnik PC, Aub JC, Brues AM (1945) The
toxic factors in experimental traumatic shock. III. Shock accompanying muscle ischemia and loss of vascular fluid. J Clin Invest 24:389–844

Keul J, Doll E, Keppler D (1969) Muskelstoffwechsel. Barth, Munich

Khan MA (1976) Histochemical characteristics of vertebrate striated muscle. A review. Fischer, Stuttgart

Kiessling WR, Ricker K, Pflughaupt KW, Mertens HG, Haubitz J (1981) Serum myoglobin in primary and secondary skeletal muscle disorders. J Neurol 224:229–233

Kindhäuser V, Eigler FW (1980) Das Tourniquet Syndrom – Ursachen und Sofortmaß-
nahmen. Notfall Med 6:129–132

Kingsley NW, Stein JM, Levensson SM (1979) Measuring tissue pressure to assess the
severity of burn-induced ischemia. Plast Recont Surg 63:404–408

Klabunde RE, Mayer StE (1979) Effects of ischemia on tissue metabolites in red(slow) and
white(fast) skeletal muscle of chicken. Circ Res 45:366–373

Klammer HL, Schulz RF (1981) Langzeitergebnisse und sozialökonomische Effizienz bei
Makroreplantation. Hefte Unfallheilkd 158:470–476

Kleinert HE, Kasdan ML (1963) Salvage of devascularized upper extremities, including
studies on small vessel anastomoses. Clin Orthop 29:29–38

Kleinert HE, Jablon M, Tsu MT (1980) An overview of replantation and results of 347 replants in 245 patients. J Trauma 20:390–398

Klenerman L, Mackie J, Chakrabarti, Brozovic M (1977) Changes in hemostatic system
after application of a tourniquet. Lancet I:970–972

Kline GD (1980) Operative experience with major lower-extremity nerve lesions, including
the lumbosacral plexus and the ischiatic nerve. In: Omer GE (ed) Management of peripheral nerve problems. Saunders, Philadelphia

Knochel JP (1976) Renal injury in muscle diseases. Perspect Nephrol Hypertens 3:129–
140

Koch B, Krüger R, Schweiberer L (1981) Pathophysiologische Folgen der Extremitätenischämie und Indikation zur Amputation. Hefte Unfallheilkd 158:677–688

Kohama A, Boyd WA, Ballinger CM, Ueda T (1971) Adenosine triphosphatase activities
of subcellular fractions of normal and ischemic muscle. J Surg Res 11:297–302

Koletsky S, Klein DE (1955) Reversibility of tourniquet shock with massive saline therapy.
Am J Physiol 182:439–442

Komatsu S, Tamai S (1968) Successful replantation of a completely cut-off thumb. Plast Recont Surg 42:374–377

Kontos HA (1971) Role of hypercapnic acidosis in the local regulation of blood flow in skeletal muscle. Circ Res 28:I98–I105

Korthals JK, Wisniewski HM (1976) Peripheral nerve ischemia. I. Experimental mode. J Neurol Sci 24:65–76

Koslowski L (1959) Autolyse-Krankheiten in der Chirurgie. Thieme, Stuttgart

Koter H, Gutschi S, Paschner O, Reschauer R (1980) Zur posttraumatischen Gefäßrekonstruktion im cruralen Bereich. 3rd Meeting of the Department of Vascular Surgery, University of Munich, November 1980

Kowanow WW, Oksman TM, Saburova LM (1968) Regionale Perfusion als Methode zur Bestimmung der Vollwertigkeit von Extremitäten vor der Reimplantation. Arch Klin Chir 322:1141–1144

Kramlova M, Pristoupil TJ, Ulrych S, Hrkal Z (1976) Stroma-free hemoglobin solution for infusion: changes during storage. Haematologia 10:365–371

Krebs B, Jensen TS, Kroner K, Nielsen J, Jorgensen HS (1985) Phantom limb phenomena in amputees seven years after limb amputation. In: Fields HL (ed) Advances in pain research and therapy, vol 9. Raven, New York

Kristen H, Eigler FW, Stock W (1970) Zur Gefahr der akuten Kaliumintoxikation nach Spätembolektomien. Langenbecks Arch Chir 327:1063–1065

Krogh A (1919a) The number and distribution of capillaries in muscles with calculations of the oxygen pressure head necessary for supplying the tissue. J Physiol 52:409–415

Krogh A (1919b) The supply of oxygen to the tissues and the regulation of the capillary circulations. J Physiol 52:457–474

Küttner H (1918) Die Verschüttungsnekrose ganzer Extremitäten. Bruns Beitr Klin Chir 112:581–600

Kunze K (1969) Das Sauerstoffdruckfeld im normalen und pathologisch veränderten Muskel. Springer, Berlin Heidelberg New York

Kuhn GG (1982) Funktionswandel nach Handverlust. Z Orthop 120:414

Kuwata N, Kawai S, Doi K (1984) Clinical and experimental studies of bone union in reimplantation of digits: a preliminary report on ischemic interval. Microsurgery 5:30–35

Lacelle PL, Weed RJ (1971) The contribution of normal and pathologic erythrocytes to blood rheology. Progr Hematol 7:1–31

Lanchow General Hospital (1973) Regeneration of veins and lymphatics after limb replantation in dogs. Chin Med J 6:77–78

Lang G, Kehr P, Jung A (1982) Unsere Erfahrungen und Spätresultate mit der Sauerbruch'schen willkürlich bewegbaren künstlichen Hand bei Arm- und Unterarmamputierten. Z Orthop 120:416

Langohr HD, Langohr U, Dieterich K, Janzig HH, Mayer K (1975) Repräsentative Enzyme des energieliefernden Stoffwechsels im normalen und denervierten M. biceps brachii, M. deltoides, M. tibialis anterior des Menschen. J Neurol 209:255–270

Lanz U (1979) Ischämische Muskelnekrosen. Springer, Berlin Heidelberg New York

Lapchinsky AG (1960) Recent results of experimental transplantation of preserved limbs and kidneys and possible use of this technique in clinical practice. Ann NY Acad Sci 87:539–571

Larcan A, Matthieu P, Helmer J, Fieve G (1973) Severe metabolic changes following delayed revascularisation: Legrain-Cormier syndrome. J Cardiovasc Surg 14:609–614

Larsson J, Bergström J (1978) Electrolyte changes in muscle tissue and plasma in tourniquet ischemia. Acta Chir Scand 144:67–73

Larsson J, Gidlöf A, Risberg B, Saugstad OD, Sahlin K, Lewis DH (1981) Total ischemia: metabolic consequences, including effects on fibrinolysis. Bibl Anat 20:588–591

Lauterjung KL, Stock W (1973) Zeitlicher Verlauf der intravaskulären Thrombozytaggregation nach 5-stündiger Ischämie einer Hundeextremität. Langenbecks Arch Chir [Suppl]:343–346

Lavine DM (1976) The failure of survival of autogenous free grafts of whole gracilis muscle in dogs. Plast Reconstr Surg 58:221–223

Lazarus-Barlow WS (1894) The pathology of the edema which accompanies passive congestion. Phil Trans R Soc Lond 185:779–817

Leaf A (1973) Cell swelling: a factor in ischemic tissue injury. Circulation 48:455–458

Lee KS (1981) Panel discussion, major limb replantation. 6th Symposium of the International Society for Reconstructive Microsurgery, Melbourne, 1981

Legros-Clark WE, Blomfield LB (1945) The efficiency of intramuscular anastomoses with observations on the regeneration of devascularized muscle. J Anat 79:15–33

Lendvay P (1981) Panel discussion, major limb replantation. 6th Symposium of the International Society for Reconstructive Microsurgery, Melbourne, 1981

Lepage GA (1946) Biological energy transformation during shock as shown by tissue analysis. J Physiol 145:267–281

Letac R, Chassaigne JP, Letac S, Beruti A (1963) Données experimentales sur la pathogénie et la prévention des troubles consecutifs à la compression musculaire ischémique. Pathol Biol 11:1028–1038

Leung PC (1981) Prolonged refrigeration in toe-to-hand transfer. Case report. J Hand Surg 6:152–153

Lewis DH (1984) Die Reaktion der Mikrogefäße des Skelettmuskels auf Blutverlust, Trauma und Ischämie. In: Hammersen F (ed) Die Mikrozirkulation des Skelettmuskels. Karger, Basel

Ley K, Arfors KE (1982) Changes in macromolecular permeability by intravascular generation of oxygen free radicals. Microvasc Res 24:25–33

Lindbom L (1983) Microvascular blood flow distribution in skeletal muscle. Acta Physiol Scand [Suppl] 525

Lindbom L, Arfors AE (1984) Über die Beziehungen zwischen der Verteilung der arteriolären Perfusion und der Kapillarströmung im Skelettmuskel. In: Hammersen F (ed) Die Mikrozirkulation des Skelettmuskels. Karger, Basel

Lindbom L, Tuma RF, Arfors KE (1980) Influence of oxygen on perfused capillary density and capillary red cell velocity in rabbit skeletal muscle. Microvasc Res 19:197–208

Linder F, Vollmar J (1965) Der augenblickliche Stand der Behandlung von Schlagaderverletzungen und ihrer Folgezustände. Chirurg 36:55–63

Lindner DJ, Miller SH, Buck DC, Demuth RJ (1985) Attempts to improve tissue survival during ex vivo storage. 30th Plastic Research Council, American Society for Plastic and Reconstructive Surgery, Portland

Little JH, Cooper C, Sarwar A, Waisman J, Fonkalsrud EW (1973) Factors influencing endothelial injury and vascular thrombosis after perfusion. J Surg Res 14:221–227

Little RA, Reynolds MJ (1976) Role of tissue fluid hyperosmolality in the pathogenesis or posttraumatic fluid loss. Br J Exp Pathol 57:387–294

Lopez-Majano V, Rhodes BA, Wagner HN (1969) Arterio-venous shunting in extremities. J Appl Physiol 27:782–785

Love BT (1978) The tourniquet. Aust NZ J Surg 48:66–70

Ludatscher RM, Hashmonal M, Monies-Chass J, Schramek A (1981) Progressing alterations in transient ischemia of skeletal muscles: an ultrastructural study. Acta Anat 11:320–327

Lundborg G (1970) Ischemic nerve injury. Scand J Plast Reconstr Surg [Suppl] 6

Lundborg G (1975) Structure and function of the intraneural microvessel as related to trauma, edema formation and nerve function. J Bone Joint Surg 57 A:938–948

Lundborg G (1977) Intraneural microvascular pathophysiology as related to ischemia and nerve injury. In: Daniel RK (ed) Reconstructive microsurgery. Little, Boston

Lundborg G (1982) Ischemic tissue injury – peripheral nerves. Scand J Plast Reconstr Surg [Suppl] 19:10–15

Lundsgard-Hansen P (1980) Synthetisches Blut. Dtsch Med Wochenschr 105:1197–1198

Lundvall J (1972) Tissue hyperosmolality as a mediator of vasodilatation and transcapillary fluid flux in exercising skeletal muscle. Acta Physiol Scand [Suppl] 379

Macfarlane MF, Spooner SJL (1946) Chemical changes in muscle during and after ischemia. Br J Exp Pathol 27:339–348

Maeiwa M, Fukumoto A, Shikata I (1970) Postmortem changes in muscles: changes in the ATP levels of muscle with time and the effects on it of chemical agents. Tokushima J Exp Pathol 17:33–40

Mäkitie J (1977) Microvasculature of rat striated muscle after temporary ischemia. Acta Neuropathol 37:247–253

Mäkitie J, Teräväinen H (1977 a) Peripheral nerve injury and recovery after temporary ischemia. Acta Neuropathol 37:55–63

Mäkitie J, Teräväinen H (1977 b) Histochemical studies of striated muscle after temporary ischemia in the rat. Acta Neuropathol 37:101–109

Mäkitie J, Teräväinen H (1977 c) Ultrastructure of striated muscle of the rat after temporary ischemia. Acta Neuropathol 37:237–245

Mailänder P, Schaller E, Schneider W, Berger A (1985) Perfusion nichtreplantierbarer Finger mit oxygenierbarer Hb-Lösung. Beitrag zur Indikationsstellung. 8th Working Conference of the DAM, Vienna

Majno G, Gilmore V, Leventhal M (1967) On the mechanism of vascular leakage caused by histamine-type mediators. Circ Res 21:833–847

Makris G, Papasoglu O, Kalakonas P, Mantinaos K, Dalainas V, Antoniadis A, Galamis N, Vrettos M (1973) Metabolic changes and late results in two cases of reimplantation of the upper limb. J Cardiovasc Surg 14:615–618

Malt RA, McKhann CF (1964) Replantation of severed arms. JAMA 189:716–722

Malt RA, Remensnyder JP, Harris WH (1972) Long-term utility of replanted arms. Ann Surg 176:334–342

Manke DA, Summer DS, Vanbeek AL, Lambeth A (1980) Hemodynamic studies of digital and extremity replants and revascularisations. Surgery 88:445–452

Marquard E (1965/66) Erfahrungen mit pneumatischen Prothesen. Verh Dtsch Orthop Ges 52:346–352

Marquard E (1975) Amputationen im Bereich der oberen Extremität. Working Conference on Emergency Trauma Care, Baden-Baden, 1975

Marquard E, Popplow K, Hillig A (1976) Psychologische Probleme in Verbindung mit Amputationen. Rehabilitation 15:174–181

Martin FR, Paletta FX (1966) Tourniquet paralysis. South Med J 59:951–953

Marty A (1973) Die Extremitäten-Replantation als gefäßchirurgischer Noteingriff. Chirurg 44:82–85

Massion WH, Blümel G (1971) Irreversibility in shock: role of vasoactive kinins. Anesth Anal 50:970–978

Mathes StJ, Nahai F (1982) Clinical application for muscle and musculocutaneous flaps. Mosby, St. Louis

Matsen FA (1980) Compartmental syndromes. Grune, and Stratton, New York

Matsuda M, Shibara H, Kato N (1978) Long-term results of replantation of 10 upper extremities. World J Surg 2:603–612

Matthias FR, Lasch HG (1981) Pathophysiologie des Schocks unter besonderer Berücksichtigung der schockspezifischen Hämostasestörung. Unfallchirurgie 7:105–111

Mau H (1969) Die ischämischen Kontrakturen der unteren Extremitäten und das Tibialis-anterior-Syndrom. Enke, Stuttgart

Mau H (1982) Kompartment-Syndrome der unteren Extremität. Z Orthop 120:202–206

Maurer PC, Heiss J, Bonke S, Lange J, Hopfner R, Duspiva W, Stock W, Bartels H, Kramann B (1979) Replantation von Gliedmaßen. Unfallheilkd 82:237–245

Maurer PC, Heiss J, Doerrler J, Burmeister W (1986) Replantation of Limbs. In: Bergan JJ (ed) Vascular surgical emergencies. Grune and Stratton, Orlando

May J (1981) Digit replantation with full survival after 28 hours of cold ischemia. Plast Reconstr Surg 67:566

May JW, Gallico GG (1980) Upper extremity replantation. Year Book Medical, Chicago (Current problems in surgery)

May JW, Chai LA, O'Brien B, Hurley JV (1978) The no-reflow phenomenon in experimental free flaps. Plast Reconstr Surg 61:256–267

Mayer RF, Eiken O, Nabseth DC (1964) Nerve regeneration in replanted canine limbs. Am J Physiol 206:1425–1421

Mazer N, Barbieri CH, Gonzalves RP (1986) Effect of different irrigating solutions on the endothelium of small arteries: experimental study in rats. Microsurgery 7:9–28

McGilvery RW (1973) The use of fuels for muscular work. In: Howald H (ed) Proceedings of the 2nd symposium on the biochemistry of exercise, Magglingen

McNamara MJ, Seaber AV, Urbaniak JR (1985) Deleterious changes in venous and arterial endothelium caused by irrigation fluids. Congress of the American Society of Reconstructive Microsurgery, Las Vegas, 1985

McNeill JF, Wilson JSP (1970) The problems of limb replacement. Br J Surg 57:365–377

Mehl RL, Paul HA, Shorey WD, Schneewind JH, Beattie EJ (1964a) Patency of the microcirculation in the traumatically amputated limb. A comparison of common perfusates. J Trauma 4:495–505

Mehl RL, Paul HA, Shorey WD, Schneewind JH, Beattie EJ (1964b) Treatment of toxemia after extremity replantation. Arch Surg 89:871–879

Meigner M, Desjars P, Malinge M, Lignon J, Nicolas F (1979) Réimplantation d'un membre au niveau de l'épaule. Anesth Analg 36:343–346

Melmon KL, Cline MJ (1967) Interaction of plasma kinins and granulocytes. Nature 213:90–92

Menger MD, Sack FU, Barker J, Meßmer K (1986) Prophylaxe des Reperfusionsschadens nach Ischämie durch Hämodilution. 2nd Congress of the German Society for Vascular Surgery, Düsseldorf, 1986

Mentha C (1959) La maladie des ligatures sans ligature ou le syndrome postanoxémique des tissus. Contribution à l'étude de la maladie de Volkmann. Lyon Chir 55:340–351

Mes TGB (1980) Improving flap survival by sustaining cell metabolism within ischemic cells. Plast Reconstr Surg 65:56–65

Meroney WH (1955) The phosphorus-to-nonprotein nitrogen ratio in plasma as an index of muscle devitalisation during oliguria. Surg Gynecol Obstet 100:309–314

Messmer K, Intaglietta M (1986) Die Bedeutung der arteriolären Vasomotion. In: Trübestein G (ed) Conservative therapy of arterial occlusive disease. Thieme, Stuttgart

Messmer K, Jesch F, Schaff J, Schoenberg M, Pielsticker K, Bonhard K (1978) Oxygen supply by stroma-free hemoglobin. In: Blood substitutes and plasma expanders. Liss, New York

Meyer V (1984) Contracture of intrinsic muscles – a problem in replantation. 5th AOA International Symposium on Limb Reconstruction – Macro- or Microsurgery? Boca Raton

Miller HH, Welch CS (1949) Quantitative studies on the time factor in arterial injuries. Ann Surg 130:428–438

Miller SH, Price G, Buck D, Neely J, Kennedy TJ, Graham WP, Davis TS (1979a) Effects of tourniquet ischemia and postischemia edema on muscle metabolism. J Hand Surg 4:547–555

Miller SH, Eyster E, Saleem A, Gottlieb L, Buck D, Graham WP (1979b) Intravascular coagulation and fibrinolysis within primate extremities during tourniquet ischemia. Ann Surg 190:227–230

Milton St (1972) Experimental studies on island flaps. II. Ischemia and delay. Plast Reconstr Surg 49:444–447

Minami S (1923) Über Nierenveränderungen nach Verschüttungen. Virchows Arch 245:247–267

Mitsuno T, Ohyanagi H, Naito R (1982) Clinical study of a new perfluorchemical whole blood substitute (Fluosol DA). Ann Surg 195:60–74

Molzberger H, Stock W, Heugel W, Welter H, Isselhard W (1977) Vergleichende Untersuchung des Energiestoffwechsels der Skelettmuskulatur von Mensch, Hund und Ratte während langfristiger Ischämie. Langenbecks Arch Chir [Suppl]:125–139

Molzberger H, Heugel E, Isselhard W (1978) Muskelstoffwechselstatus beim Tourniquet-Syndrom der Ratte nach Anwendung des Proteaseninhibitors Aprotinin. Arzneimittel Forsch 3:394–397

Monies-Chass I, Hashmonai M, Hoerer D, Kaufmann Th, Steiner E (1977) Hyperbaric oxygen treatment as an adjuvant to reconstructive vascular surgery in trauma. Injury 8:274–277

Montagnani CA, Simeone FA (1953) Observations on the liberation and elimination of myohemoglobin and of hemoglobin after release of muscle ischemia. Surgery 34:169–185

Moore CD, Cardea JA (1977) Vascular changes in leg trauma. South Med J 70(2):1285–1286

Moore DH, Nickerson JL, Powell AE, Marks G (1951) A study of the transfer of serum proteins into tissue injured by tourniquet. Proc Soc Exp Biol Med 77:706–706

Morrison WA, McO'Brien B, McLeod AM (1977) Major limb replantation. Orthop Clin 8:343–348

Mortensen WW, Hargens AR, Gershuni DH, Crenshaw AG, Garfin StR, Akeson WH (1985) Long-term myoneural function after induced compartment syndrome in the canine hind limb. Clin Orthop Rel Res 195:289–293

Morton JH, McReynolds G, Stradford HT (1969) Reimplantation of the upper arm: possibilities and problems. J Trauma 9:3–16

Moxley RT, Griggs RC, Vangelter V, Theile R, Herr BE (1978) Effects of denervation and wasting on skeletal muscle blood flow in man. Neurology 28:400

Mubarak SJ, Owen CA, Hargens AR, Garetto LP, Akeson WH (1978) Acute compartment syndromes: diagnosis and treatment with the aid of the wick catheter. J Bone Joint Surg 60 A:1091–1095

Mumenthaler M, Schliack H (1982) Läsionen peripherer Nerven. Thieme, Stuttgart

Muramatsu I, Takahata N, Usui M, Ishii S (1985) Metabolic and histologic changes in the ischemic muscles of replanted dog legs. Clin Orthop Rel Res 196:292–299

Myrhage R, Eriksson E (1984) Die Anordnung der Gefäße in verschiedenen Typen von Skelettmuskeln. In: Hammersen F (ed) Die Mikrozirkulation des Skelettmuskels. Karger, Basel

Myrhage R, Hudlicka O (1978) Capillary growth in chronically stimulated adult skeletal muscle as studied by intravital microscopy and histological methods in rabbits and rats. Microvasc Res 16:73–90

Nabseth DC, Mayer RF, Deterlin RA (1966) Experimental basis of limb replantation. In: Welch CE (ed) Advances in surgery, vol 2. Chicago

Nachbur B, Horber F, Gänger KH, Descoeudres C (1983) Die metabolische Bedrohung nach Rekonstruktion der arteriellen Strombahn bei schwerster Muskelischämie. Helv Chir Acta 50:749–751

Nakahara M (1971) The effect of a tourniquet on the kinin-kininogen system in blood and muscle. Thromb Diath Haemorrh 26:264–274

Narayan KK, Im MJ, Manson PN, Hoopes JE (1985) Mechanism and prevention of ischemia/reperfusion injury in skin flaps. 30th Plastic Research Council, American Society of Plastic Reconstructive Surgery, Portland, 1985

Nasseri M, Voss H (1973) Late results of successful replantation of upper and lower extremities. Ann Surg 177:121–125

Nathansson IT, Nutt AL, Pope A, Zamecnik PC, Aub JC, Brues AM, Kety SS (1945) The toxic factors in experimental traumatic shock. I. Physiologic effects of muscle ligation in the dog. J Clin Invest 24:829–834

Newmann RJ (1984) Metabolic effects of tourniquet ischaemia studied by nuclear magnetic resonance spectroscopy. J Bone Joint Surg 66-B:434–440

Nghiem DG, Boland JP (1980) Four-compartment fasciotomy of the lower extremity without fibulectomy. A new approach. Am Surg 46:414–417

Nunley JA, Koman LA, Urbaniak JR (1981) Arterial shunting as an adjunct to major limb revascularisation. Ann Surg 193:271–273

O'Brien B McC (1977) Microvascular reconstructive surgery. Churchill, Edinburgh

O'Brien, B McC (1981) St. Vincents hospital clinical program, major limb replantation. 6th Symposium of the International Society for Reconstructive Microsurgery, Melbourne, 1981

O'Brien B McC, McLeod AM (1976) Replantation surgery of limbs. In: Daniller AJ (ed) Symposium on microsurgery. Mosby, St. Louis

Ochoa J, Fowler TJ, Gilliat RW (1972) Anatomical changes in peripheral nerves compressed by a pneumatic tourniquet. J Anat 113:433–455

O'Connel TX, Sanchez M, Mowbray JF, Fonkalsrud EW (1974) Effects on arterial intima of saline infusion. J Surg Res 16:197–203

O'Donovan MJ, Rowleson A, Taylor A (1976) The perfused isolated human limb: an assessment of its viability. J Physiol 256:27P–28P

Oestrup LT (1983) Bone transplantation by microvascular anastomoses. 1st International symposium on microsurgery in reconstructive and plastic surgery, Jena, 1983

Ohshiro T, Mukai K, Kosaki G (1980) Prevention of hemoglobinuria by administration of haptoglobin. Res Exp Med 177:1–12

Omer GE (1981) Nerve, neuroma, and pain problems related to upper limb amputation. Orthop Clin North Am 12:751–762

Onji Y, Murai Y, Tamai S, Hashimoto T, Yamaguchi T, Ariyama A, Tsujimoto A (1963) Experimental surgery on resuscitation and reunion of amputated or nearly amputated leg. Plast Reconstr Surg 31:151–165

O'Regan S, Fong JSC, Drummond KN (1979) Renal injury after muscle extract infusion in rats. Absence of toxicity with myoglobin. Experientia 35:805–806

Osterman AL, Heppenstall B, Sapega AA, Katz M, Chance B, Sokolow D (1984) Muscle ischemia and hypothermia: a bioenergetic study using ^{31}phosphorus nuclear magnetic resonance spectroscopy. J Trauma 24:811–817

Paletta FX (1968) Replantation of the amputated extremity. Ann Surg 168:720–727

Paletta FX, Willmann V, Ship AG (1960) Prolonged tourniquet ischemia of extremities. J Bone Joint Surg 42 A:945–950

Paletta FX, Shedhadi SJ, Mudd JG, Cooper T (1962) Hypothermia and tourniquet ischemia. Plast Reconstr Surg 29:531–538

Pappenheimer JR (1948) Effects of osmotic pressure of the plasma proteins and other quantities associated with the capillary circulation in the hindlimb of cats and dogs. Am J Phys 152:471–491

Patterson S, Klenerman L (1979) The effect of pneumatic tourniquets on the ultrastructure of skeletal muscle. J Bone Joint Surg 61:178–183

Paul HA, Mehl RL, Schneewind JH, Beattie EJ (1965) Shock in replantation and crush syndrome: a comparison of the clinical evolution and the results of treatment. J Trauma 5:349–357

Pausescu E, Proinov F, Chirvasie R, Fagaranasu D, Dabuleanu L, Dudugian ML (1976) Early biochemical disorders in hindlimb muscles following femoral artery stenosis in dogs. Eur Surg Res 8:504–514

Pausescu E, Proinov F, Chirvasie R, Fagaranasu D, Dudugian ML (1977) Early biochemical disorders in the hindlimb muscles following femoral artery stenosis in dogs: protein and electrolyte metabolism. Z Exp Chir 10:216–225

Peacock EE, Madden JW, Trier WC (1969) Transfer of median and ulnar nerves during early treatment of forearm ischemia. Ann Surg 169:748–756

Pennig D, Brug E (1982) Die prognostische Bedeutung der muskulären pH-Registrierung in der Replantationschirurgie. Hefte Unfallheilkd 158:467–470

Perri GC, Gorini P (1952) Uraemia in the rabbit after injection of cristalline myoglobin. Br J Exp Pathol 33:440–444

Persson NH, Erlansson M, Svensjö E, Takolander R, Bergquist (1985) Postischemic macromolecular permeability increase is reduced by repeated ischemia. Soc Int Chir, Schwabe, Basel, Abstract p. 676

Petterson S, Hansson R, Jonsson O, Lundstam S, Schersten T (1983) Effect of free-radical inhibition on renal circulation after ischemia. 13th International Meeting of the Nordic Microvascular Group, Geilo, 1983

Pfannkuch F, Schnoy N (1979) Verbleib des blutgastransportierenden Fluorkohlenwasserstoffs Fluorocarbon 43 im Organismus bei parenteraler Anwendung im Tierversuch. Anaesthesist 28:511–516

Pfannkuch F, Schnoy N, Öhlschlegel Ch, Wilson C (1981) Vergleichende morphologische Untersuchungen nach parenteraler Anwendung von Fluosol 43, DA 20 und DA 35 in Tierexperimenten. International symposium of oxygen carrying colloidal substitutes, Mainz, 1981

Piza H, Millesi H, Meissl G, Walzer R, Mandl H, Freilinger G, Holle J, Frey M (1983) Kritische Betrachtungen der Makroreplantation. Congress of the Austrian Society of Plastic Surgery, Linz, 1983

Plyley MJ, Groom AC (1975) Geometrical distribution of capillaries in mammalian striated muscles. Am J Physiol 228:1376–1383

Pongratz D (1976) Differentialdiagnose der Erkrankungen der Skelettmuskulatur. Thieme, Stuttgart

Pope A, Zamecnik PC, Aub JC, Brues AM, Dubos RJ, Nathansson JT, Nutt AL (1945) The toxic influence of the bacterial flora, particularly *Clostridium Welchii*, in exsudates of ischemic muscle. J Clin Invest 24:856–863

Presta M, Cipollini T, Mazzocchi C, Cuccinello C, Ragnosti G (1981) Hematochemical modifications after muscle ischemia. Influence of hypothermia. In: Brunelli G (ed) Ischemia and reimplantation. Liviana, Padua

Proctor KG, Duling BR (1982) Oxygen free radicals and local control of striated muscle blood flow. Microvasc Res 24:77–86

Quigley JT, Popich GA, Lanz UB (1981) Compartment syndromes of the forearm and hand. Clin Orthop 161:247–251

Rahmer H, Durst J, Schubert GE (1977) Correlation between local oxygen tension in muscle tissue and survival time in tourniquet shock. Circ Shock 4:35–40

Ramirez MA, Marcos Duque G, Hernandez L, Londono A, Cadavid G (1967) Reimplantation of limbs. Plast Reconstr Surg 40:315–324

Ravin HA, Denson JR, Jensen H (1954) Electrolyte swifts and electrocardiographic changes during tourniquet shock in rats. Am J Physiol 178:419–426

Reichert FL (1926) The regeneration of the lymphatics. Arch Surg 13:871–881

Reichert FL (1931) The importance of circulatory balance in the survival of replanted limbs. Bull Johns Hopkins Hosp 49:86–93

Rembs E, Isselhard W, Cordes G, Hohlfeld T (1984) Cardioplegic solution HTP (Bretschneider) fails to protect ischemic limbs and to influence tourniquet shock. Eur Surg Res 16:110–111

Reneman RS (1968) The anterior and the letal compartment syndrome of the leg. Proefschrift, Monton, Amsterdam

Reneman RS, Slaaf DW, Lindbom L, Tangelder GJ, Arfors KE (1980) Muscle blood flow disturbances produced by simultaneously elevated venous and total muscle tissue pressure. Microvasc Res 20:307–318

Renkin EM (1971) The nutritional-shunt-flow hypothesis in skeletal muscle circulation. Circ Res 28:21–25

Reznik M (1970) Satellite cells, myoblasts, and skeletal muscle regeneration. In: Mauro A (ed) Regeneration of striated muscle and myogenesis. Excerpta Medica, Amsterdam

Reznik M, Hansen JL (1969) Mitochondria in degenerating and regenerating skeletal muscle. Arch Pathol 87:601–608

Rhea WG, Foster JH (1961) A study of the influence of heparin and low-molecular-weight dextran on tourniquet palsy. Surg Forum 12:436–438

Rhodes GR, Newell JC, Shah D, Scovill W, Tauber J, Dustin RE, Powers SR (1978) Increased oxygen consumption accompanying increased oxygen delivery with hypertone mannitol in adult respiratory distress syndrome. Surgery 84:490–497

Richards RR, Seaber AV, Urbaniak JA (1985) Chemically induced vasospasm: the effect of ischemia, vessel occlusion and adrenergic blockade. Plast Reconstr Surg 75:238–244

Richt G, Wendt P, Wölfl I, Vassiliou I, Mittelmeier T, Blümel G (1984) Die Wirkung eines Sauerstoffträgers bei der initialen Perfusion von Extremitäten vor Replantation. Metabolische und hämodynamische Parameter im Tierexperiment. Langenbecks Arch Chir [Suppl] 364:535

Riede UN, Mittermayer Ch, Friedburg H, Sandritter W (1981) Pathologie und Pathophysiologie des Kreislaufschocks mit besonderer Berücksichtigung der Schocklunge. Unfallchirurgie 7:97–104

Risberg B, Smith L, Sternberg B (1985) Prevention of edema formation in the perfused lung preparation by oxygen radical scavengers. Eur Surg Res 17:230–236

Ritland D, Butterfield W (1973) Extremity complications of drug abuse. Am J Surg 126:639–648

Robinson AJ, Holcroft JW, Olcott C, Blaisdell FW (1975) Pulmonary and coagulation changes in tourniquet shock. J Surg Res 19:65–70

Roder JD, Lehmann-Horn F, Buchner U, Hölscher M, Ehrhardt W (1985) Neurophysiologische Parameter zur Beurteilung der Extremitätenischämiebelastbarkeit und Reversibilität von Ischämiefolgen. Langenbecks Arch Chir Suppl 227–230

Romanul FCA, Hogan EL (1965) Enzymatic changes in denervated muscle. Arch Neurol 13:263–273

Romanul FCA, Pollock A (1969) The parallelisms of changes in oxidative metabolism and capillary supply of skeletal muscle fibers. In: Locke S (ed) Modern neurology. Little, Boston

Romanul FCA, van der Meulen JP (1967) Slow and fast muscles after cross-innervation. Arch Neurol 27:387–402

Romanul FCA, Sreter FA, Salmons S, Gergely J (1974) The effect of a changed pattern of activity on histochemical characteristics of muscle fibers. In: Milhorat AT (ed) Exploratory concepts in muscular dystrophy. Excerpta Medica, Amsterdam

Romanus M (1977) Microcirculatory reactions to local pressure-induced ischemia. Acta Chir Scand [Suppl] 479

Romeis B (1968) Mikroskopische Technik, 16th edn. Oldenbourg, Munich

Rompe G, Niethard FU (1982) Probleme des Haltungs- und Bewegungsapparats als Folge der Amputation. Z Orthop 120:121

Roome NW, Wilson H (1935) Experimental shock. The effect of extracts from traumatized limbs on the blood pressure. Arch Surg 31:361–370

Rorabeck CH (1980) Tourniquet-induced nerve ischemia: an experimental investigation. J Trauma 20:280–286

Rosen H, Slivjak MJ, McBrearty FX (1985) Preischemic flap washout and its effect on the no-reflow phenomenon. Plast Reconstr Surg 76:737–747

Rosenkrantz JG, Sullivan RC, Welch K, Miles JS (1967) Replantation of an infant's arm. N Engl J Med 276:609–612

Ross G, White FN, Brown AW, Kolin A (1966) Regional blood flow in the rat. J Appl Physiol 21:1273–1275

Rossi F, Bellavite P, Berton G, Grzeskowiak M, Papini E (1985) Mechanism of production of toxic oxygen radicals by granulocytes and macrophages and their function in the inflammatory process. Pathol Res Pract 180:136–142

Rotter W (1958–59 a) Über die postischämische Insuffizienz überlebender Zellen und Organe, ihre Erholungszeit und die Wiederbelebungszeit nach Kreislaufunterbrechung. Thoraxchirurgie 6:107–124

Rotter W (1958/59 b) Über die Pathologie der postischämischen Erholungsperiode. Berichte der Oberhessischen Gesellschaft für Natur- und Heilkunde, University Library, Frankfurt

Rowland LP, Fahn S, Hirschberg E, Harter DH (1964) Myoglobinuria. Arch Neurol 10:537–562

Rubinstein NA, Kelly AM (1978) Myogenic and neurogenic contributions to the development of fast- and slow-twitch muscles in rat. Dev Biol 62:473–485

Ruby LK (1978) Acute traumatic amputation of an extremity. Orthop Clin 9:679–692

Rüter A, Burri C (1982) Grenzindikation des Erhaltungsversuchs und Indikation zur primären Amputation bei Verletzungen. Z Orthop 120:612

Russell RC (1985) Fillet of sole flap for immediate lower-limb stump reconstruction. Europ Plast Surg Workshop, Zürs

Russell RC, O'Brien B McC, Morrison WA, Pamamull G, McLeod A (1984) The late functional results of upper-limb revascularisation and replantation. J Hand Surg 9A:623–633

Saldeen T (1979) The microembolism syndrome: a review. Almquist, Stockholm

Saar FvG (1913) Über Blutleere der unteren Körperhälfte. Ergeb Chir Orthop 6:1–46

Salesses M, Moussu P, Aupecle M (1962) Deux observations „princeps" de section traumatique quasi complète du bras suivie d'opération restauratrice et de conservation de membre. Acad Chir 88:930–940

Sanderson RA, Foley RK, McIvor GWD, Kirdaldy-Willis WH (1975) Histological response of skeletal muscle to ischemia. Clin Orthop 113:27–35

Santangelo ML, Usberti M, Disalvo E, Belli G, Romano R, Sassarolo C, Zooti G (1982) A study of the pathology of the crush syndrome. Surg Gynecol Obstet 154:372–374

Santavirta S, Luoma A, Arstila AU (1979) Morphological and biochemical changes in striated muscle after experimental tourniquet ischemia. Res Exp Med 174:245–251

Saunders JH, Sissons HA (1953) The effect of denervation on the regeneration of skeletal muscle after injury. J Bone Joint Surg 35 B:113–124

Savitsky JP, Doczi J, Black J, Arnold JD (1978) A clinical safety trial of stroma-free hemoglobin solution. Clin Pharm Ther 23:73–80

Scharnagel E (1986) Extremitätenreplantation unter besonderer Berücksichtigung flankierender Massnahmen. Handchirurgie 18:275–288

Scherer H, Piger A, Maurer P, Mack D (1973) Verminderung des postischämischen Gliedmaßenoedems nach Arterienrekonstruktion durch den Proteinasenhemmer Trasylol. In: Huber A (ed) Probleme des geschwollenen Beins. Brunner, Bern

Schindler HG, Pennig D, Schlake W, Schönleben K, Brug E (1981) Fluosol 43 als Dauerperfusat zur Überbrückung der Anoxiezeit an abgetrennten Extremitäten im Tierexperiment. International symposium of oxygen carrying colloidal substitutes, Mainz, 1981

Schlagetter K, Zimmermann H (1956) Experimentelle Untersuchungen über Blut- und Knochenmarksveränderungen nach vorübergehender Ischämie der unteren Körperhälfte. Beitr Pathol Anat 116:574–593

Schlenker JB (1982) The effect of hypothermia and tissue perfusion on extended myocutaneous flap viability. Plast Reconstr Surg 70:453–454

Schmalbruch H (1970) Die quergestreiften Muskelfasern des Menschen. Erg Anat Entw Gesch 43, Springer, Berlin Heidelberg New York

Schmalbruch H (1980) Entwicklung, Untergang und Regeneration von Skelettmuskelfasern. Dtsch Med Wochenschr 105:614–617

Schmalbruch H (1981) Wie die Katze den Vogel fängt. Dtsch Med Wochenschr 106:1040–1042

Schmid-Schönbein H, Fischer T, Driessen G, Rieger H (1979) Microcirculation. In: Hwang NHC (ed) Qualitative cardiovascular studies. University of Baltimore Press, Baltimore

Schneider M, Hauck H, Förster H, Hübner K (1976) Tierexperimentelle morphologische Untersuchungen über die Auswirkung stroma-freier Lösungen einfachen und polymerisierten Hämoglobins auf Leber und Niere. Verh Dtsch Ges Pathol 60:194–199

Schneider M, Hauk H, Förster H, Hübner K (1978) Morphologische Untersuchungen der Organveränderungen nach Infusion verschiedenartiger perfluorierter Kohlenwasserstoffe bei Ratten. Verh Dtsch Ges Pathol 62:312–315

Schnitzer W, Stock W (1973) Die Erhöhung des osmotischen Gewebedrucks als Ursache des postischämischen Extremitätenoedems. Langenbecks Arch [Suppl]:21–24

Schoenberg MH, Fredholm BB, Hohlbach G (1985) Changes in acid-base status, lactate concentration and purine metabolites during reconstructive aortic surgery. Acta Chir Scand 151:227–233

Schröder JM (1982) Pathologie der Muskulatur. Springer, Berlin Heidelberg New York

Schubert GE, Durst J, Rahmer H (1976) Morphologische Befunde im Tourniquet Schock. Res Exp Med 169:155–167

Schwiegk H (1942) Schock und Kollaps. Klin Wochenschr 34:741–749

Scully RF, Shannon JM, Dickersin GR (1961) Factors involved in recovery from experimental skeletal-muscle ischemia produced in dogs. Am J Pathol 39:721–737

Seddon HJ (1966) Volkmann's ischemia in the lower limb. J Bone Joint Surg 48 B:627–636

Seddon HJ (1972) Surgical disorders of the peripheral nerve. Churchill, London

Sehgal LR, Rosen AL, Noud G, Sehgal HL, Gould SA, Dewoskin R, Rice CL, Moss GS (1981) Large-volume preparation of pyridoxylated hemoglobin with high p-50. J Surg Res 30:14–20

Selverstone B, White JC (1956) Autonomic recovery. In: Woodhall B (ed) Peripheral nerve regeneration, study of 3656 World War II injuries. Vet Ad Med Monogr US Government Printing Office, Washington

Shaftan GW, McAlvanah MJ (1976) Experience with replantation of hands and arms. In: Daniller AJ (ed) Symposium on microsurgery. Mosby, St. Louis

Shah DM, Powers SR, Stratton HH, Newell JC (1981) Effects of hypertonic mannitol on oxygen utilisation in canine hindlimbs following shock. J Surg Res 30:593–601

Shandall M, Hallett B, Williams G, Young HL (1985) Reperfusion injury of the colon and oxygen radical production. Soc Internat Chir. Schwabe, Basel, p 159

Shaw RS (1963) Treatment of the extremity suffering near or total severance with special consideration of the vascular problem. Clin Orthop 29:56–71

Shehadi SI, Paletta FX, Cooper T (1961) Effect of hypothermia on circulatory responses in the canine hindlimb after tourniquet ischemia. Surg Forum 12:466–468

Sheridan WW, Matsen FA, Krugmire RB (1977) Further investigations on the pathophysiology of the compartmental syndrome. Clin Orthop 123:266–270

Sherman RA, Sherman CJ, Parker L (1984) Chronic phantom and stump pain among American veterans: results of a survey. Pain 18:83–94

Shires GT, Cunningham JN, Bauer CRF, Reeder SF, Illner H, Wagner IY, Mauer J (1972) Alterations in cellular membrane function during hemorrhagic shock in primates. Ann Surg 176:288–295

Siebert H, Messner H, Pannike A, Vontin H (1975a) Beobachtungen zur Tourniquetischämie: das Verhalten der Thrombozytenzahl und des Fibrinogens nach 3-stündiger Extremitäten-Tourniquetischämie bei splenektomierten und nicht-splenektomierten Hunden. Monatsschr Unfallheilkd 78:551–557

Siebert H, Messner H, Pannike A (1975b) Beobachtungen zur Tourniquetischämie: Untersuchungen über den Einfluß von Milz und Fraktur auf Blutzellaggregation, ATP-Gehalt und freie Fettsäuren nach dreistündiger Extremitäten-Tourniquetischämie bei Hunden. Monatsschr Unfallheilkd 78:558–563

Silin PJ, Strulowitz JA, Wolin MS, Belloni (1985) Absence of a role for superoxide anion, hydrogen peroxide and hydroxyl radical in endothelium-mediated relaxation of rabbit aorta. Blood Vessels 22:65–73

Sinagowitz E, Rahmer H, Rink R, Görnadt L, Kessler M (1973) Local oxygen supply in intra-abdominal organs and in skeletal muscle during hemorrhagic shock. Adv Exp Med Biol 37 A:505–511

Sixth People's Hospital, Shanghai (1967) Reattachment of traumatic amputations. A summing up of experience. China Med J 5:392–402

Sixth People's Hospital, Shanghai (1975) Hyperbaric oxygen therapy in replantation of severed limbs. Chin Med J I:197–204

Skalak TC, Schmid-Schönbein W, Zweifach BW (1984) New morphological evidence for a mechanism of lymph formation in skeletal muscle. Microvasc Res 28:95–112

Skinner SN, Costin JC (1971) Interactions between oxygen, potassium and osmolality in regulation of skeletal muscle blood flow. Circ Res 28 I:73–85

Smahel J (1982) Effect of a deproteinized blood extract on the recovery of blood circulation in an ischemic skin lesion. Br J Exp Pathol 63:177–183

Smith AR, van Alphen B, Faithful NS, Fennema M (1985) Limb preservation in replantation surgery. Plast Reconstr Surg 75:227–237

Snyder CC (1963) Autoplantation of extremities. Clin Orthop 29:113–122

Snyder CC, Knowles RP (1977) Autotransplantation of limbs. In: Converse JM (ed) Reconstructive plastic surgery. Saunders, Philadelphia, pp 2178–2196

Snyder WH (1982) Vascular injuries near the knee: an updated series and overview of the problem. Surgery 91:502–506

Solonen K, Hjelt L (1968) Morphologic changes in striated muscle during ischemia. Acta Orthop Scand 39:13–19

Solonen K, Tarkanen L, Närvänen S, Gordin R (1968) Metabolic changes in the upper limb during tourniquet ischemia. Acta Orthop Scand 39:20–32

Sommerlad BC, McGrauther DA (1978) Resurfacing the sole: long-term follow-up and comparison of techniques. Br J Plast Surg 31:107–116

Spalteholz W (1888) Die Verheilung der Blutgefäße im Muskel. Abhandl K S Ges Wiss 14:509–527

Spence RJ, Rhodes BA, Wagner HN (1972) Regulation of arteriovenous anastomotic and capillary blood flow in the dog leg. Am J Physiol 222:326–332

Stalker CG, McEwan AJ, McAledingham J (1973) The effect of increased oxygen in acute limb ischemia. Br J Surg 60:144–148

Stallone RJ, Blaisdell FW, Cafferata HT, Levin SM (1969) Analysis of morbidity and mortality from arterial embolectomy. Surgery 65:207–217

Staples D, Topuzlu C, Blair E (1969) A comparison of ATP levels in hemorrhagic and endotoxin shock in the rat. Surgery 66:883–885

Steinau HU (1985) Großreplantation und Postischämiesyndrom. Habilitationsschrift, University of Frankfurt

Steinau HU, Elert O, Schneider M (1979) Die Verlängerung der warmen Ischämietoleranzzeit an abgetrennten Extremitäten. 3rd Haemoglobin Colloquium. Biotest, Frankfurt

Steinau HU, Elert O, Schneider M (1980) Prolongation of the ischemia tolerance of amputated extremities by a stroma-free hemoglobin solution. Thorac Cardiovasc Surg 28:35

Steinau HU, Elert O, Schneider M (1981) Experimentelle Untersuchung zur Skelettmuskelperfusion mit stroma-freier Hämoglobinlösung unter Ischämiebedingungen. Handchirurgie 13:149–151

Stenger RJ, Spiro D, Scully RE, Shannon JM (1962) Ultrastructural and physiologic alterations in ischemic skeletal muscle. J Pathol 40:1–20

Stiegler H, Nees S, Klug M, Böck M (1985) Untersuchungen zur Antithrombogenität der Venenwand und deren Beeinflussung durch Thrombose. 1st Congress of the German Society for Vascular Surgery, Munich

Stingl J (1970) Zur Frage der Gefäßversorgung der Skeletmuskulatur. Acta Anat 76:488–504

Stingel J (1971) Zur Ultrastruktur des terminalen Gefäßbetts der Skelettmuskulatur. Acta Anat 80:255–272

Stingl J, Stembera O (1974) Distribution and ultrastructure of the initial lymphatics of some skeletal muscles in the rat. Lymphology 7:160–168

Stipa S, Cavallaro A, Privitera L (1967) Treatment of shock following prolonged ischemia of the limbs. J Cardiovasc Surg 8:529–534

Stock W (1974) Tierexperimentelle Untersuchungen zur Ursache der hohen Letalität nach Wiederherstellung der Durchblutung akut ischämisch geschädigter Extremitäten. Habilitationsschrift, University of Cologne

Stock W, Eigler FW (1969) Wirkung eines Proteaseninhibitors auf das Tourniquet-Syndrom der Ratte. Z Ges Exp Med 151:64–73

Stock W, Themann H, Isselhard W (1974) Konservierung der Skelettmuskulatur des Hundes durch Perfusion mit Magnesium-Aspartat. In: Frey R (ed) Elektrolyte und Spurenelemente in der Intensivmedizin. De Gruyter, Berlin

Stock W, Biertz P, Geppert E, Isselhard W (1976) Die Konservierung von Hundeextremitäten durch hypotherme Perfusion. Langenbecks Arch Chir [Suppl]:308–311

Stone AM, Stein T, Lafortune J, Wise L (1979) Renal vascular effects of stroma and stroma-free hemoglobin. Surg Gynecol Obstet 149:874–876

Stoner HB (1958a) Studies on the mechanism of shock: the influence of environment on the changes in oxygen consumption, tissue temperature and blood flow produced by limb ischemia. Br J Exp Pathol 39:251–277

Stoner HB (1958b) Studies on the mechanism of shock: the quantitative aspects of glycogen metabolism after limb ischemia in the rat. Br J Exp Pathol 39:635–651

Stoner HB, Green HN (1948) Bodily reactions to trauma: the effect of ischemia on muscle protein. Br J Exp Pathol 29:121–132

Streuli HK (1970) Oberschenkelreplantation nach Bahnunfall. Helv Chir Acta 37:237–240

Strock PE, Majno G (1969a) Microvascular changes in acutely ischemic rat muscle. Surg Gynecol Obstet 129:1213–1224

Strock PE, Majno G (1969b) Vascular response to experimental tourniquet ischemia. Surg Gynecol Obstet 129:309–318

Strock PE, Majno G, Diethelm AG (1968) Protection of vascular patency of the ischemic dog limb by various perfusate solutions. In: Norman JC (ed) Organ perfusion and preservation. Appleton, New York

Strohfeld P (1973) Das isoliert perfundierte Hinterbein der Ratte als Modell zur Untersuchung des Muskelstoffwechsels. Res Exp Med 162:7–16

Stroinska-Kusiowa B (1979) Microangiographic studies of denervated, reinnervated and hypertrophied muscles of rats. J Neurol 220:65–70

Stuhler T, Schneider D (1982) Oberschenkelamputationen, eine Langzeitverlaufsanalyse. Z Orthop 120:612

Su ChT, Im MJ, Hoopes JE (1982) Tissue glucose and lactate following vascular occlusion in island skin flaps. Plast Reconstr Surg 70:202–205

Sullivan P (1986) Ischemia-induced synthesis of prostaglandins in man. 31st Plast Res Council ASPRS, Norfolk

Sunderland S (1972) Nerve and nerve injuries. Churchill, London

Sunder-Plassmann L, Sinagowitz E, Rink R, Dieterle R, Messmer K, Kessler M (1973) The local oxygen supply in tissue of abdominal viscera and of skeletal muscle in extreme hemodilution with stroma-free hemoglobin solution. Adv Exp Med Biol 37:395–400

Suzuki M, Penn J (1966) The effect of therapeutic agents upon the microcirculation during general hypothermia. Surgery 60:807–878

Swartz WM, Cha CJM, Ambler M, Clowes GHA (1976) Prolonged ischemia in the replanted rat leg: a biochemical and morphologic study with microvascular techniques. Surg Forum 27:565–568

Swartz WM, Cha CJ, Clowes GHA, Randall HT (1978) The effect of prolonged ischemia on high-energy phosphate metabolism in skeletal muscle. Surg Gynecol Obstet 147:872–876

Taheri SA, Heffner R, Williams J, Lazar L, Elias S (1984) Muscle changes in venous insufficiency. Arch Surg 119:929–931

Tamai S (1982) Twenty years' experience of limb replantation – review of 293 upper-extremity replants. J Hand Surg 7:549–556

Tamai S, Tatsumi Y, Shimizu T, Hori Y, Okuda H, Takita T, Sakamoto, Fukui A (1977) Traumatic amputation of digits: the fate of remaining blood. J Hand Surg 3:13–21

Tamai S, Hori Y, Tatsumi Y, Okuda H, Nakamura Y, Sakamoto H, Takita T (1979) Major limb, hand, and digital replantation. World J Surg 3:17–28

Tangelder GJ, Slaaf DW, Reneman RS (1984) Die Mikrozirkulation des Skelettmuskels und ihre Beziehung zu Änderungen des transmuralen und des Perfusionsdrucks. In: Hammersen F (ed) Die Mikrozirkulation des Skelettmuskels. Karger, Basel

Tauber A, Wendt P, Mittelmaier T, Beisbarth H, Maurer P, Blümel G (1981) Initiale Spülung von Replantaten mittels Fluosol 43: metabolische und hämodynamische Untersuchungen. International Symposium on oxygen-carrying colloidal blood substitutes, Mainz, 1981

Taylor GI (1977) Free nerve transfer. In: Daniel RK (ed) Reconstructive microsurgery. Little, Boston

Telepneva VJ (1973) Metabolism of NAD and NADP in normal and denervated muscles. In: Kakulas BA (ed) Basic research in myology. Excerpta Medica, Amsterdam

Thomason PR, Matzke HA (1975) Effects of ischemia on the hind limb of the rat. Am J Physiol Med 54:113–131

Thompson WW, Gilbert MD, Campbell S (1959) Studies in myoglobin and hemoglobin in experimental crush syndrome in dogs. Ann Surg 149:235–242

Threllfall CJ, Stoner HB (1957) Studies on the mechanism of shock: the effect of limb ischemia on the phosphates of muscle. Br J Exp Pathol 28:339–356

Thulesius O, Silvertsson R (1973) Ischämisches und postischämisches Oedem. In: Hubert A (ed) Probleme des geschwollenen Beins. Brunner, Bern

Thulborn KR (1981) ^{31}P NMR studies of energy metabolism and tissue pH in the ischemic rat leg. Biochem Soc Trans 9:237–238

Torii S, Harii K, Ohmori K (1979) Experimental study of ischemia time influencing free flap survival. Chir Plast 4:225–233

Tountas CP, Bergman RA (1977) Tourniquet ischemia: ultrastructural and histochemical observations of ischemic human muscle and of monkey muscle and nerve. J Hand Surg 2:31–37

Trump BF, Mergner WJ, Kahn MW, Saladino AJ (1976) Studies on the subcellular pathophysiology of ischemia. Circulation 53:I17–I29

Trunkey DD, Illner H, Wagner IY, Shires GT (1973) The effect of hemorrhagic shock on intracellular muscle action potentials in the primate. Surgery 74:241–250

Tsai TM (1981) Panel on major limb replantation. 6th Symposium of the International Society for Reconstructive Surgery, Melbourne, 1981

Tsai TM, Jupiter JB, Serratoni F, Seki T, Okubo K (1982) The effect of hypothermia and tissue perfusion on extended myocutaneous flap viability. Plast Reconstr Surg 70:444–452

Tsai TM, Doden O, Buffer G, Firrel J, Takahashi F (1985) Prevention of ischemic damage to muscle by perfluorocarbon emulsion. 8th Symposium of the International Society Reconstructive Microsurgery, Paris, 1985

Tuma RF, Childs CM, Intaglietta M, Afors KE (1975) Microvascular flow pattern in the tenuissimus muscle. Bibl Anat 13:151–152

Unseld H, Aderhold B, Stähler D, Schubert GE, Schneider K (1976) Die Belastbarkeit der Nieren des Zwergschweins mit stromafreier Hämoglobinlösung. Proceedings of the Congress on Blood Transfusion and Haematology, Biotest Institute, Frankfurt

Usui M, Ishif S, Muramatsu I, Takahata N (1978) An experimental study on replantation toxemia. J Hand Surg 3:589–596

Usui M, Ishii S, Muramatsu I (1983) An experimental study on the effect of fluorocarbon on the preservation of free skin flaps in the rabbit. Clin Orthop 175:273–279

Van der Meer C, Valkenburg PW, Ariens AT, Vanbenthem RMJ (1966) Cause of death in tourniquet shock in rats. Am J Physiol 210:513–525

Veicsteinas A, Comande S (1981) Nerve and muscle viability after tourniquet and cuff ischemia in hypothermia. In: Brunelli G (ed) Ischemia and reimplantation. Liviana, Padua

Vilkki SK (1985) Freie Zehenübertragung auf den Unterarmstumpf nach Handgelenksamputation – eine moderne Alternative zur Krukenberg-Operation. Handchir Mikrochir Plast Chir 17:92–97

Vitali M, Robinson KR, Andrews BG, Harris EE (1978) Amputations and prostheses. Baillière Tindall, London

Volkmann R (1893) Über die Regeneration des quergestreiften Muskelgewebes beim Menschen und Säugetier. Beitr Pathol Anat 12:297–324

Von Volkmann R (1881) Die ischämischen Muskellähmungen und Kontrakturen. Zentralbl Chir 8:801–814

Wählby L, Dahlbäck LO, Sjöström M (1978) Achilles tendon injury. Acta Chir Scand 144:359–369

Wang SH, Young KF, Wei JN (1981) Replantations of severed limbs – clinical analysis of 91 cases. J Hand Surg 6:311–318

Warburg O (1948) Wasserstoffübertragende Fermente. Saenger, Berlin

Weeks RS (1968) The crush syndrome. Surg Gynecol Obstet 127:369–375

Weinberg H, Song Y (1983) The no-reflow phenomenon and its modification: an analysis by perfusion fluorometry. Annual Convention of the American Society of Plastic and Reconstructive Surgery, Dallas, 1983

Weissman G, Korchak HM, Perez HD, Smola JE, Goldstein IM (1979) Leucocytes as secretary organs of inflammation. In: Weissman G (ed) Advances in inflammation research, vol 1. Raven, New York, pp 95–112

Welch WD, Rose DM, Carlson R (1982) Reduced hemoglobin as an inhibitor of human polymorphonuclear leucocyte bacterial killing. Surgery 91:75–80

Welter H, Stock W, Hermann G (1974) Immunelektrophoretische Untersuchungen der Proteinverteilung im postischämischen Oedem des Hundes im Vergleich zu Serum und Lymphe. Res Exp Med 163:47–62

White JC (1969) Nerve regeneration after replantation of severed arms. Ann Surg 170:715–719

White JC, Selverstone B (1956) Pain and related phenomena including causalgia. In: Woodhall B (ed) Peripheral nerve regeneration. Vet Adm Monogr US Government Printing Office, Washington

Wiesmann U, Kaspar U, Mumenthaler M (1969) Necrosis and regeneration of the tibialis anterior muscle in rabbit. Biochemical changes. Arch Neurol 21:373–380

Wildbolz U (1970) Die Regeneration des denervierten Skelettmuskels nach ischämischer Nekrose. Acta Anat 77:238–258

Williams GR (1966) Replantation of amputated extremities. Monogr Surg Sci 3:53–83

Williams JR, Jefferson D, Gilliat RW (1980) Acute nerve compression during limb ischemia. J Neurol Sci 46:199–207

Willms-Kretschmer K, Majno G (1969) Ischemia of the skin. Am J Pathol 54:327–353

Wilson H, Roome NW (1936) The effects of constriction and release of an extremity. An experimental study of the tourniquet. Arch Surg 32:334–345

Winkler W, Baumgartner R (1981) Myoelektrische Armprothesen. Enke, Stuttgart

Winninger AL (1972) Biopathological disturbances in the revascularisation stage of ischemic limbs. J Cardiovasc Surg 14:640–648

Wissing H, Schmitt-Neuerburg KP (1982) Diagnose und Differentialdiagnose des Kompartmentsyndroms, Unfallheilkd 85:133–143

Wollenberger A, Ristau O, Schoffa G (1960) Eine einfache Technik der extrem schnellen Abkühlung großer Gewebestücke. Pflugers Arch 270:399–402

Woodhall B, Beebe GW (1956) Peripheral nerve regeneration. Vet Adm Monogr US Government Printing Office, Washington

Worman LW, Darin JC, Kritter AE (1965) The anatomy of a limb replantation failure. Arch Surg 91:211–215

Yakovlev NN (1973) The role of sympathetic nervous system in the adaptation of skeletal muscles to increased activity. In: Howald H (ed) Proceedings of the 2nd international symposium on the biochemistry of exercise, Magglingen

Yokoyama H, Hirakawa S, Kida K, Satch E, Inui T (1979) Blood flow distribution in microcirculatory beds of the striated muscle of dogs' hind limbs. Influences of acute venous congestion and hemorrhagic hypotension. 2nd World Congress on Microcirculation, La Jolla, 1979

Yong LC (1980) Regeneration of lymphatic vessels in the ear of guinea pigs. J Pathol 131:209–219

Yoon JO (1986) The role of metal ions in ischemia/reperfusion injury in skin flaps. A site-specific mechanism. 31st Plastic Research Council, American Society of Plastic and Reconstructive Surgery, Norfolk, 1986

Yoshioka T, Sugimoto T, Ukai T, Oshiro T (1985) Haptoglobin therapy for possible prevention of renal failure following thermal injury: a clinical study. J Trauma 25:281–287

Yoshizu T, Katsumi M, Tajima T (1978) Replantation of untidily amputated finger, hand and arm: experience of 99 replantations in 66 cases. J Trauma 18:194–200

Zamecnik PC, Aub JC, Brues AM, Kety SS, Nathanson JT, Nutt AL, Pope A (1945) The toxic factors in experimental traumatic shock. V. Chemical and enzymatical properties of muscle exsudate. J Clin Invest 24:850–855

Zdeblick TA, Shaffer JW, Field GA (1985) An ischemia-induced model of revascularisation failure of replanted limbs. J Hand Surg 10[Am]:125–131

Zierler KL (1965) The skeletal muscle circulation. In: Mills LC (ed) Shock and hypotension. Grune and Stratton, New York

Zimmermann H, Springer N (1966) Vergleichende experimentelle enzymbiochemische, histochemische und morphologische Untersuchung an der ischämisch geschädigten Skelettmuskulatur des Kaninchens. Z Pathol 75:187–206

Zrubecky G (1977) Derzeitige Grenzen moderner Technologie bei Prothesen an Arm und Hand. 18th Symposium of the German Society of Hand Surgery, Erlangen, 1977

Zucman J (1960) Studies on the vascular connections between periosteum, bone and muscle. Br J Surg 48:324–328

Zwank L (1981) Therapeutische Möglichkeiten bei der offenen Gefäßverletzung. Hefte Unfallheilkd 158:693–701

Zwank L, Eckert P (1983) Ergebnisse von Beinreplantationen. Langenbecks Arch Chir [Suppl] 361:945

Zwank L, Hertel P, Schweiberer L (1980a) Replantationen – Funktion und soziale Aspekte. Dtsch Arztebl 45:2657–2670

Zwank L, Hertel P, Schweiberer L, Alayan H (1980b) Funktionelle Ergebnisse nach Replantationen. Unfallheilkd 148:565–575

Zweifach SS, Hargens AR, Evans KL, Smith RK, Mubarak SJ, Akeson WH (1980) Skeletal muscle necrosis in pressurized compartments associated with hemorrhagic hypotension. J Trauma 20:941–947

Subject Index

Blalock, A. 2
Brooks, B. 22
Bywaters, E. 2

Capillaropathy, ischemia induced 83, 24ff, 67ff, 86
Carrel, A. 1
Compartment syndrome
  clinical conditions 30
  critical closing pressure 31
  late sequalae 32
  reperfusion injury 30f, 89, 92
  treatment 31f, 92
Critical repair phase 29

Declamping phenomenon 47, 53ff, 85ff, 92

Energy rich phosphagens, measurements 84

Fiber type
  distribution 16, 17, 89
  capillary structure 14, 18
  metabolism and ultrastructure 18
  regulatory mechanisms 16ff
Fluorocarbons, complications 77f, 79f
Frankenthal, L. 2, 35
Free muscle transplantation 28

Hackradt, A. 2, 35
Halsted, W. 1
Hemoglobin solution
  endothelial lining 58
  muscle protection 62ff, 81, 87, 90
  product description 41
  radiolabeled 49, 56, 57, 87
  side effects 65, 81, 87, 88
Historical review 1
Höpfner, E. 1
Hyperbaric oxygenation 79

Ischemia, definition 9
Ischemia-induced injury
  bone 10
  capillary system 24ff, 67ff, 58ff

cartilage 10
connective tissue 10
dermis and subcutaneous tissue 9
intracellular lesion 20ff
lymphatic system 11
muscle, smooth 15, 19, 23, 30
muscle, striated 18ff, 27ff, 89
tolerance 9

Jeger, E. 1
Jianu, J. 1

Legenda aurea 1
Legrain-Cormier-syndrome 33
Low flow perfusion 84
Lymphatic system 11, 12
  regeneration following amputation 11, 12
  toxic products 39

Malt, R. 2, 74
Major limb replantation
  complications 4, 8, 34, 23ff, 37ff
  rehabitational aspects 3
  statistical frequency 2, 3, 74
  success rate 8, 75
Minor limb replantation 75
Muscle, smooth 15, 19, 23, 30, 87
Muscle, striated
  anatomical and physiological basis 14
  arterio-venous anastomoses 16, 31
  capillary perfusion 15
  cell metabolism 18
  edema, interstitial, intracellular 20, 21, 59, 83
  individual vulnerability 19
  ischemia induced myopathy 20, 59, 66ff, 86
  ischemia tolerance 19, 21, 22, 66ff, 89
  lymphatic system 11f
  point of no return 21
  postischemic membrane insufficiency 21, 66ff, 86, 89
  regeneration 22, 27, 28, 59ff, 92
  regulation of blood flow 15, 16

R. T. Manktelow

Microvascular Reconstruction

Anatomy, Applications and Surgical Technique

With Section on Paediatrics by R. M. Zuker

Foreword by G. I. Taylor

Illustrated by K. Finch

1986. 288 figures. XIII, 221 pages.
ISBN 3-540-15271-7

The use of microvascular techniques has increased greatly over the last fifteen years. This book is aimed at experienced surgeons and trainees as a 'when, what, and how to'-guide to microvascular reconstructive surgery. It discusses the selection, anatomy, and surgical technique of a spectrum of free tissue transfers, divided into two parts. The first section covers the surgical anatomy and technique involved in elevating each of the free tissue transfers, and the second discusses the applications of these transfers to reconstruction in three specific areas where reconstructive microsurgery has made its major contributions: the head and neck, the upper extremity, and the lower extremity. Written for the most part by a single surgeon, this highly practical reference work is purposely dogmatic with the aim of providing useful solutions to patients' problems.

Springer-Verlag
Berlin Heidelberg New York
London Paris Tokyo

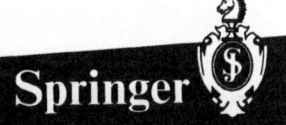

Springer

B.-D. Katthagen, Homburg/Saar

Bone Regeneration with Bone Substitutes

An Animal Study

1987. 101 figures. X, 159 pages.
ISBN 3-540-17425-7

Congenital and acquired bone defects constitute a central problem of traumatology and orthopedics. In order to cure these defects it is often necessary to fill up the bones operatively with suitable substances. For this purpose, bone transplants are preferred. Recently, so-called bone substitutes (collagen, gelatine, bone matrix, calcium phosphate, hydroxyapatite) have also been recommended. Following an introductory presentation of bone regeneration and transplants, these substitutes are discussed here in a comprehensive survey of the literature. The author has carried out comparative histomorphometric examinations of bone regeneration under the influence of the abovementioned bone substitutes. Particular attention is given to the significance of mineral substance such as hydroxyapatite, which will undoubtedly find a place in bone surgery owing to its outstanding bioactivity and biocompatibility. The implants examined are also of significance for maxillofacial surgery and dentistry. The histologic techniques in undecalcified bone preparations and in histomorphometry are presented in a special chapter.

Springer-Verlag
Berlin Heidelberg New York
London Paris Tokyo

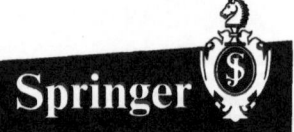

Springer